D0729422

Chiropractic:

Compassion and Expectation

Terry A. Rondberg, D.C.
and
Timothy J. Feuling

The
Chiropractic
Journal

Chiropractic:
Compassion and Expectation

Published by:
The Chiropractic Journal

Library of Congress Catalog Number: 98-74388

ISBN: 0-9647168-6-0

Printed in the United States of America
1 2 3 4 5 6 7 8 9 10 11 12

Photos of B. J. Palmer and D. D. Palmer used with permission of Palmer College of Chiropractic Archives.

Cover concept and photos used with permission of Sherman College of Straight Chiropractic.

Cover by: C. Michael Rhodes
Book design by: Marlan Publishing Group, Ltd.

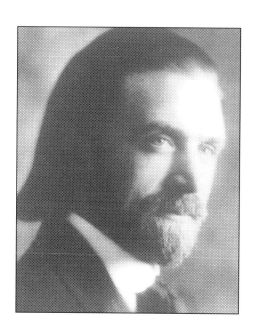

We dedicate this book
to the man who is known as the
"Developer of Chiropractic,"
Bartlett Joshua (B.J.) Palmer.
His dedication not only ensured that chiropractic would
survive as a distinct and separate health care system for the
benefit of all humanity, but as a personal inspiration and
model of what all of us can strive to achieve.

"To be great is to be misunderstood."

— B.J. Palmer

WHAT THE READERS ARE SAYING...

"Chiropractic: Compassion and Expectation is a must read gift to every Principled Chiropractor for everyone of their patients. The authors have in a clear, concise and interesting fashion explained chiropractic as it is, an integral necessity for a well-adjusted society."

Luis E. Ocon, D.C.
Salinas, California

"Chiropractic: Compassion and Expectation answers many questions for the prospective and already enthusiastic chiropractic patient. It answers the basics; what is it, how can it help my family and me? It also gives patients the ammunition to defend their decision to utilize chiropractic. It does what all good books should do—causes people to think."

John A. Hofmann, D.C., F.I.C.A.
Allen Park, Michigan

"Chiropractic: Compassion and Expectation is an exciting and informative book about the truth in health care, and the position in which chiropractic lends itself to those who wish to experience the highest level of life and health. The authors have written a book that I feel is a 'must read' for all chiropractors and their patients. Every reader will walk away with a deeper appreciation for the chiropractic principles and the innate laws of healing."

Ronald J. Oberstein, D.C.
San Diego, California

"Compassion is the understanding of the sufferings of others. The authors are very aware of the chiropractic condition and the need to serve more. This book shares my dedication to family health. This book is 'the' chiropractic document."

James R. Milliron, D.C., F.I.C.A.
Yakima, Washington

"We all owe the authors a vote of thanks for writing Chiropractic: Compassion and Expectation. This book gives us a fresh and comprehensive perspective of what the chiropractic profession is all about. Every doctor owes it to themselves to share this information with the rest of the world."

Herbert Ross Reaver, D.C.
Pisgah, Ohio

"This book is unique. It answers many questions that people ponder before committing to chiropractic care. Should I see a D.C.? What will my first visit be like? Chiropractors practice differently, what are these differences? This book answers questions that no other text answers."

Joseph W. Accurso, D.C.
Miami, Florida

"This book is for anyone who desires a full understanding of the chiropractic practice objective. When the people we serve are fully informed they will intelligently recommend and properly refer others with a higher degree of confidence."

Wesley S. Mullen, Jr., D.C., F.I.C.A.
Mountaintop, Pennsylvania

About the Authors

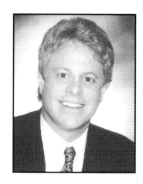

Dr. Terry A. Rondberg is a prominent leader in the chiropractic profession. After graduating from Logan College of Chiropractic in 1975, he began his private practice, helping thousands of patients from his offices in St. Louis, Missouri and Phoenix, Arizona. In 1986, he founded *The Chiropractic Journal*, a successful, widely-read international monthly focusing on public information and political action concerning chiropractic.

In 1989, Dr. Rondberg founded the World Chiropractic Alliance, a non-profit "watchdog" organization which has led the movement to protect consumers' rights to name chiropractic as their first choice in health care. Dr. Rondberg is also president of Chiropractic Benefit Services, the fastest growing chiropractic professional liability program in the United States.

Reflecting both the depth of his knowledge and the enthusiasm of his convictions, Dr. Rondberg is in demand as a speaker at chiropractic conventions and seminars. A prolific writer, he is the author of many professional and popular articles and books.

With his gift for writing and speaking about chiropractic, Dr. Rondberg has helped inform millions of individuals around the world about the philosophy, art and science of chiropractic.

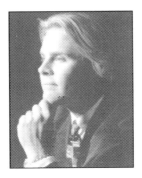

Timothy J. Feuling has lived the "chiropractic lifestyle" since 1990. He majored in finance at Arizona State University and continues to study the intricacies of business.

Mr. Feuling has studied the art, philosophy and science of chiropractic and therefore understands the importance of informing the public about the devastating effects of vertebral subluxation. He has devoted his life to serving the chiropractic profession and all those people who have yet to discover chiropractic care.

Mr. Feuling is Vice President of the World Chiropractic Alliance and specializes in helping doctors reach their potential through the proper choice of insurance and related services. He also serves as Vice President of Chiropractic Benefit Services Professional Liability Program.

Foreword

by Christopher Kent, D.C., F.C.C.I., President of the Council on Chiropractic Practice

The revolution in health care is underway. A study in the Journal of the American Medical Association reports that people are seeking health care that is "congruent with their own values, beliefs, and philosophical orientations toward life and health."

The chiropractic profession is at the leading edge in health care reform. As the largest drugless health care profession, and the second largest healing art, the chiropractic profession has the vision, commitment, and resources to fill a vital need in society.

Dr. Terry Rondberg and Timothy Feuling have made an important contribution to this process with the publication of "Chiropractic: Compassion and Expectation." This book promises to serve as a valuable resource for any person seeking chiropractic care. It addresses concerns and controversies head-on, in a professional and understandable way.

This book clearly explains the objectives of chiropractic care, and what a patient seeking chiropractic services may expect. It clarifies the role of chiropractic in the health care system, establishing clearly that chiropractic is not an alternative therapy. Rather, chiropractic represents a separate, distinct, and necessary element in everyone's quest for health.

The World Health Organization defines health as "Optimum physical, mental, and social well being, and not merely the absence of disease or infirmity." This is the goal of the doctor of chiropractic — working to eliminate interference with a person's innate potential for wholeness.

Victor Hugo wrote that there is nothing more powerful than an idea who's time has come. I must respectfully disagree. More powerful than the idea itself is the individual who has the passion, commitment, and skill to make the idea a reality. Chiropractic is an idea who's time has come. This book is your guide to making it a reality in your life.

Rondberg and Feuling have produced this book to enable you to live a longer, happier, and more productive life. Read it carefully, and discover how chiropractic care may benefit you. Share it with others, so they can enjoy the benefits of a life that expresses their optimal potential for health and happiness.

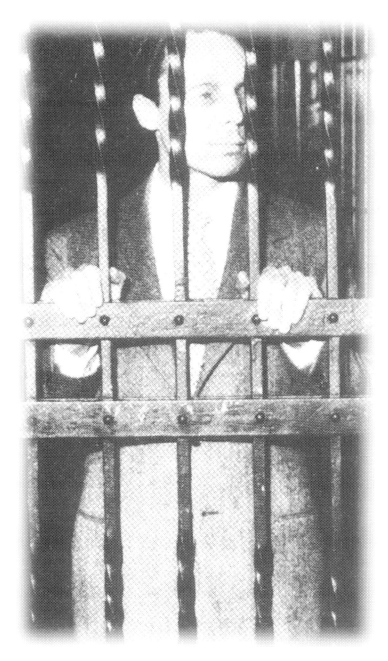

Dr. Herb Reaver is one of the chiropractic profession's most honored pioneers. His courage and dedication despite numerous arrests for trumped-up charges remain an inspiration to doctors of chiropractic around the country.

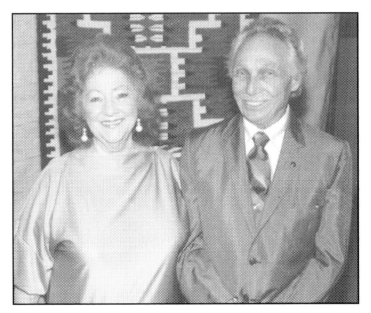

Considered one of the elder statesmen of the profession he so valiantly defended for most of his life, Dr. Herb Reaver (shown here with his lovely wife Millie) were honored by the author in a special tribute held in Phoenix, Arizona, in 1991.

Dr. Herbert Ross Reaver (Doc), went to jail 13 times in 11 years rather than admit to the false charge that he was practicing medicine without a license. Doc and Millie Reaver sacrificed so much for the evolution of the chiropractic profession.

B.J. Palmer wrote him in jail, "I love you Herbie, because you love the things I love. If chiropractic had 1,000 men like you, we could lick the world, and add one million years a day to millions of people, and what a world that would be to live in!"

The Reaver's contribution to the profession were not very widely known among the younger generation of chiropractors until recently in 1991. Dr. Terry and Cindy Rondberg invited Doc and Millie to be honored for a lifetime of contributions and sacrifices they made to the chiropractic profession. Since then, the Reavers have gained well-deserved celebrity status.

Table of Contents

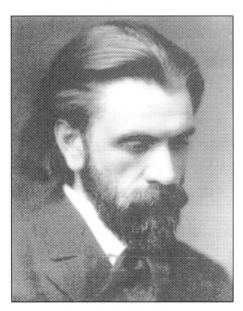

B.J.'s last printed words:

Time always has and always will perpetuate those methods which better serve mankind. Chiropractic is no exception to that rule. My illustrious father placed this trust in my keeping, to keep it pure and unsullied or defamed. I pass it on to you unstained, to protect as he would have you do. As he passed on, so will I. We admonish you to keep this principle and practice unadulterated and unmixed. Humanity needed then what he gave us. You need now what I give you. Out there in those great open spaces are multitudes seeking what you possess.

The burdens are heavy; responsibilities are many; obligations are providential; but the satisfaction of traveling the populated highways and byways, relieving suffering and adding millions of years to lives of millions of suffering people, will bring forth satisfaction and glories with greater blessings than you think. Time is of the essence.

May God flow from above-down His bounteous strengths, courage and understanding to carry on; and may your Innates receive and act on that free flow of Wisdom from above-down; inside-out... for you have in your possession a Sacred Trust. Guard it well.

Chapter 1

EXPECTATION AND HEALTH

Doctors of chiropractic are extremely fortunate. They get to combine two of the greatest professions in the world: health care and teaching. Most people don't think about chiropractors as teachers, but the good ones spend almost as much time educating their patients as they do caring for them.

That's because understanding wellness and being healthy can't be separated. To be healthy, you have to learn how your body operates and how best to keep it well. That includes learning what to expect when you seek out various health care and medical practitioners.

While there are many books written about what you can expect when you go to medical doctors — from glowing reports of medical "miracles" to documented accounts of the failures of modern medicine — there are few books which explain, in detail, what you can expect when you visit a doctor of chiropractic. Yet, with two of every five people in the United States using alternative health care, including chiropractic, it's a topic of growing importance.

Of course, many people just walk into a chiropractic

office without knowing anything about chiropractic or what it can do for them. Most of them leave happy and healthier, but they seldom get the maximum benefit from this incredible health care field. Sadly, some of them, who enter with an inaccurate or unrealistic expectation, leave frustrated and unsatisfied.

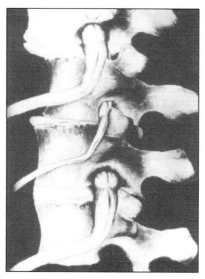

This is one type of vertebral subluxation (spinal nerve interference) — the "silent killer."

That's where chiropractic education comes in.

Whenever you enter a chiropractic office, the doctor has an opportunity to educate you about the benefits of regular spinal care. The doctor makes sure you understand that the purpose for care is to examine your spine and see if the vertebrae — the interlocking bones that make up the spinal column — are correctly aligned.

If not, it could mean you are subluxated, which interferes with your normal nerve flow, since the nerve fibers pass through the openings in the bones. If an opening is restricted, the nerve impulses may be altered as well and that will prevent your body from expressing normal function. The doctor should then explain to you that he or she does not diagnose disease or treat your ailments. The doctor's purpose is not to suppress your symptoms or cure your illnesses.

However, the doctor's going to give you the most important help possible — a subluxation-free spine. Without interference, your body will be free to do the rest!

It is quite common in a chiropractic office for patients to bring in their entire family for chiropractic care. Most patients feel healthier with each visit and they want their spouses, parents, and children to get healthier, too.

That's why Dr. Gerald Smith of Florida wasn't at all surprised when one of his long-time patients, Al Crenshaw, referred his brother Charles to his office.

Al had originally come to Dr. Smith because he was having back pain after an accident at work. During the exam, the doctor detected several subluxations, which could have been caused by the accident, or could have existed even before the accident occurred.

He started Al on a series of chiropractic adjustments and his body responded quickly, giving him the chance for his back injury to heal naturally.

Al also found himself feeling healthier in other ways, and said he had more energy and vitality than he'd had in a long time. He no longer had his regular colds and bouts with flu during the winter, and his allergies were lessening.

He was convinced that chiropractic deserved the credit, so he came in every week for a wellness visit. "Just to be on the safe side," he'd always tell Dr. Smith.

❊ ❊ ❊

WANTING PAIN RELIEF

When his brother Charles started getting bad headaches and muscle pains in his neck, Al recommended that he come to see Dr. Smith. Charles arrived at the office looking a bit skeptical, and started to describe in detail how his headaches felt.

Dr. Smith stopped him mid-sentence and began to explain that he didn't "treat" headaches. He was going to give him the new patient orientation about spinal nerve interference, but Charles cut him short by saying his brother had explained all that to him.

The doctor said, "I should have given him the session anyway, but we were very busy that week and, assuming his brother had told him the basics, I went right to the examination."

After reviewing his spinal X-ray and other tests, Dr. Smith detected a subluxation in his upper spine, close to where the skull rests on the spinal column, which is called the upper cervical region. Dr. Smith told him he'd need to come back for more adjustments before they could be sure the spinal nerve interference had been corrected and his body was "reshaped" to the proper spinal position.

Charles did return, and again started talking about his headaches. They hadn't stopped, he complained, and the muscle soreness in his neck was just as bad. Once more, the doctor tried to explain about spinal nerve interference and once more he said, "Yeah, I know. Al told me all about that. But I'm here for my headaches."

Dr. Smith gave Charles another adjustment. "I could tell

from feeling his spine that there was improvement, but it would take additional visits to make sure the adjustment held," he explained, "so I set up another appointment with him."

Unfortunately, Charles never returned. When Al came in a week or so later, Dr. Smith asked him how his brother was, and why he hadn't kept his appointment.

"He said he didn't think chiropractic worked," Al told him reluctantly. He still got a headache after the second adjustment and he decided to go to a medical doctor. They have him on painkillers now, but that's not helping too much. He's so groggy from the pills he can't even drive half the time."

Dr. Smith sighed. Obviously, Charles just didn't "get it." He looked at Al and was struck by how two people — in this case, two brothers — could have completely different attitudes about chiropractic.

The odd thing was, he had given them both the same level of care. He examined them both the same way, and specifically adjusted them. Yet, one was completely satisfied with chiropractic and realized that it had contributed a great deal to his health. The other was just as completely dissatisfied with chiropractic and would never experience any improved function after receiving regular chiropractic care.

**Knowledge is knowing a fact.
Wisdom is knowing what to do
with that fact.   — B.J. Palmer**

❖ ❖ ❖

THE EFFECT OF EXPECTATION

What was the big difference between these two very similar people?

For one thing, the doctor had taken the time to educate Al about the real purpose of chiropractic and the devastating impact of vertebral subluxations on his life and health. He understood that chiropractic wasn't going to treat or cure his back pain — only his own body's inner wisdom could do that. Only chiropractic adjustments could make sure his body wasn't ravaged by vertebral subluxations.

Al understood this and accepted the fact that his body would work better if it had a healthy nerve supply. He knew that if he specifically wanted to treat back pain, he would have to seek out a different kind of doctor and get treated while he continued to have his subluxations corrected.

In his case, the body's inner wisdom was perfectly capable of eliminating the back pain by itself, once his spinal nerve interference was corrected.

Charles was a different matter. He had never grasped the principles of chiropractic. He came to Dr. Smith wanting a cure for his headaches. He wanted him to figure out what was causing them, diagnose his condition, and treat him for that particular problem.

He didn't really want to get healthier, he wanted to get rid of his headaches. He was looking for a cure and when he didn't get one, he was disappointed and frustrated. Unfortunately, he ended up resorting to medical treatment which, according to his brother, was doing him more harm than good. Their expectations about chiropractic made the

6

critical difference in their satisfaction.

That's not at all surprising. Our expectations often have a big influence on the outcome of anything.

Take dieting, for example. Let's say you are overweight and decide to cut your calorie intake by 500 calories a day. If you expect to lose 10 pounds a week, you're going to be very frustrated at the end of a couple of weeks. Chances are, you'll get discouraged and stop dieting altogether. This is generally what happens when your expectations aren't met.

But the real failure isn't with your diet plan — it's with your expectation. Losing 10 pounds a week is unrealistic (not to mention unhealthy!). You're setting yourself up for failure and disappointment with such unrealistic expectations. Without truly understanding the way the human body works, you make it impossible to succeed.

Don't feel too badly if this kind of thing has happened to you — it happens to all of us. In fact, not long ago, it happened to us too, in a completely different way.

❖ ❖ ❖

GETTING A FATAL ERROR MESSAGE

Our office had been struggling along with a slow, old computer system for far too long and we finally made the decision to invest in a new, super-fast system, complete with a huge hard drive, lots of memory, and a multi-media sound system.

We had visions of speeding through every task without a glitch. Within the first week, we had loaded up at least two dozen programs — everything from spreadsheets to graphic design programs.

But then we started having problems. The keyboard would lock up. The Windows crash alerts were becoming more frequent. Even the desktop icons were moving around as though they had a mind of their own. We were convinced we'd bought a bad system.

The computer was possessed by some evil spirit or — at the very least — had been infected by a virus. Ultimately, like many other computer users, we blamed it all on Bill Gates.

Our first step was to run down to the computer software store and buy a program that would supposedly "fix" these problems and eliminate the error messages. We loaded it up and figured our troubles would be solved. They weren't. In fact, the computer locked up the first time we tried to run this utility program.

Finally, we called a tech support representative, who came out and examined the computer. Patiently, he explained that he was going to check out the software first since most computer problems could be traced to the programs we load up.

We asked if he knew of any other utility programs that could fix the problem and get rid of those annoying error messages. He said that would add more problems to the computer and wasn't the answer. He needed to look at it from the inside to see what the situation was.

We stepped back and decided to let him do his job. He changed some settings and booted up the machine. It crashed — again. He changed a few other things. We got another "fatal error" message. By this time, we were getting impatient. Why couldn't he fix it the first time?

But we let him try again. Once he'd given the file another "adjustment" the computer seemed to run fine. Of course, we weren't convinced, but when we didn't have another problem for the next few weeks, we had to admit he was right.

It was only much later that we realized we had done exactly what Charles Crenshaw had done. We had gone to a computer "doctor" wanting him to put something into the machine — the electronic version of a prescription — to fix everything. We didn't realize that the root cause of the difficulties was something that had interfered with the normal functioning of the computer.

Adding another program wasn't going to fix it. When the cause of the interference was corrected (in this case, it had something to do with mysterious IRQ settings) the system ran smoothly.

Had we understood better how the computer worked, and carried more realistic expectations about what the technician would do, we could have saved ourselves a lot of anxiety. Of course, it might have been worse. Like Charles, we could have decided to let our expectations dictate our actions and insisted on yet another utility program. But that wouldn't have solved the problems.

Normally, we hesitate to compare the human body to a computer. That's like comparing the sun to a light bulb. In this case, the comparison helps to make a point. Sometimes, our bodies don't work right. They "crash" and give out error messages.

In our desire to get rid of the error messages, we call on a medical doctor expecting to be given a magic pill that will make everything okay. We're more concerned with getting rid of the error messages than we are with making the computer work right.

If we go to our chiropractor with at least a basic understanding of how our bodies work, and with a realistic view of what we can expect, we'll end up not only healthier but more satisfied as well.

> # It's what we learn after we think we know it all that counts.
>
> ## — B.J. Palmer

❖ ❖ ❖

REALISTIC EXPECTATION LEADS TO SATISFACTION

Luckily, most doctors of chiropractic do a good job of educating their patients. As a result, most patients have a realistic expectation of how they will benefit from their care program and most are very satisfied with the results.

In fact, according to a study conducted in 1991 by the Gallup organization, eight of every ten chiropractic patients were satisfied with the care received and they felt that most of their expectations were met. Even the Gallup pollsters knew that our satisfaction level is directly related to our expectations.

More than 25 million people visit a doctor of chiroprac-

tic each year, making chiropractic the second largest primary health care profession in the world. If they are to leave
their D.C.'s office feeling satisfied with the care they've
received, they have to know what to expect in the first place.

If they go in expecting the doctor to diagnose or treat
their diseases, they are bound to be disappointed, since
that's not what chiropractic is for. On the other hand, if they
go realizing that their health depends on a good nerve supply — and the chiropractor's job is to eliminate interference
to that supply — then they will leave feeling confident about
their choice.

Why should this matter to the doctor of chiropractic?
After all, with more than 25 million patients (and more being
added each year) there are plenty to go around. Yet, most
D.C.s spend a lot of valuable time making sure their patients
are well educated and taking an active role in their own
health.

There are many reasons why patient satisfaction is so
important to most chiropractors. First of all, the vast majority of D.C.s chose their profession because of a strong desire
to help others. Many were chiropractic patients themselves,
and experienced first hand the power of the adjustment.
Some had been sickly as children, or injured as adults. They
tried to find medical answers, but failed to achieve health
until they found chiropractic.

Now, these doctors want to offer that same "miracle" to
others. Their **compassion** is their driving force, and they
know they won't be able to help patients if the patients don't
understand why they are there.

If they go away thinking chiropractic doesn't work
because it didn't live up to an unrealistic expectation, they will

11

never know how much it could have improved their lives.

Dr. Smith will always feel a little guilty when he thinks about Charles Crenshaw, because he didn't make sure the patient clearly understood the purpose of chiropractic and what he could reasonably expect from care.

As a result, he left before his body had a chance to improve from the adjustments he was receiving. Hopefully, his brother might be able to convince him to return for chiropractic care!

Of course, chiropractors have another very real concern. If patients are not satisfied and leave care prematurely, they often visit medical doctors. While that's not always avoidable, it can very frequently be the start of a course of unnecessary medical treatment including drugs and surgery. Chiropractors do everything in their power to help their patients with conservative chiropractic care first, using medicine only as a last resort when the body cannot heal itself without intervention.

On a strictly practical note, chiropractors also need to protect themselves from patients who have an unrealistic expectation about what chiropractic care can and will do for them. Occasionally, a patient will go to a chiropractor thinking the doctor is going to perform full-body, medical diagnosis and either treat the disease or refer him or her to a medical specialist.

If that doesn't happen, the patient could feel cheated and wrongfully sue the doctor for malpractice, particularly if a medical condition was later discovered by a medical doctor. "You should have diagnosed my cancer... my diabetes... my heart problem," they complain, not realizing that a chiropractor does not diagnose disease.

For all these reasons, doctors of chiropractic have a very strong motivation for wanting to care for their patients with the utmost compassion, but also to make sure they have a realistic expectation about chiropractic's role.

We've written this book to help patients — and all those who may become patients — better understand chiropractic and its place in the health care system, and to clearly show what one can expect from chiropractic — and why it is the most important element of a person's health care program!

After you've finished reading this book, you will know far more about how your body works, why subluxation correction is so important, and what to expect from a chiropractor. You will understand why your chiropractor does not offer full-body medical diagnosis or disease treatment, and what the courts have said on the subject.

Finally, you'll understand why your doctor of chiropractic may ask you to sign a "Terms of Acceptance" form stating that you fully understand the true scope of chiropractic and have a realistic expectation about the care you will receive from your D.C.

You'll also read about other patients whose personal case histories have helped illustrate the various points we needed to make in this book.

In essence, this book is about you, and all the more than 25 million people who know (or are learning) how chiropractic wellness care can help them live happier, healthier and more productive lives with improved function.

Chapter 2

WHERE IT ALL STARTED

I t's not surprising that many people have a wrong idea about what chiropractic is all about. For more than 100 years, since it was first developed into a unique health care profession in this country, it has been misunderstood and misrepresented.

Partly this was because it was seen as a threat to the supremacy of the medical profession. Medical doctors, at the turn of the century, were enjoying a tremendous surge in popularity.

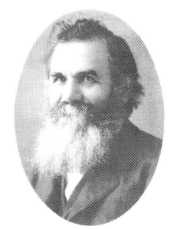

Daniel David Palmer (D.D.)

Our society adored everything scientific and technological and the medical profession — with its new chemicals, gadgets and instruments — was admired by the nation. Medical doctors didn't want any other health care profession rocking the boat.

When a lay healer named Daniel David (better known today as D.D. Palmer) began getting excellent results by "adjusting" a person's spine by applying force in a specific manner to the verte-brae, M.D.s were at first curious. A few even attended classes held by D.D. and later by his son Bartlett Joshua (B.J.) Palmer.

But medical doctors didn't like what the Palmers and the new generation of chiropractors were teaching. They were telling students that the best "physicians" in the universe were the patients themselves — that the human body had an innate intelligence which kept it constantly striving to achieve better health. If the body was allowed to work without interference, they said, it would reach and maintain its highest possible level of function.

This smacked of some kind of "hocus pocus" to the medical doctors who were willing only to believe in scientific evidence they could weigh and measure. They could remove a heart from a corpse and examine it. They could put cells under a microscope and study them. But they couldn't "see" or even prove the exis-tence of this "innate intelligence." The world, they had concluded, was merely an accident of evolution and every movement in it was random.

Physicists today, particularly those studying quantum physics have taken a 180-degree turn in scientific thought: nothing in this universe is truly random.

Actually, the "proof" was all around those skeptical M.D.s, but they either couldn't or didn't want to see it. The world definitely was a product of millions of years of evolution, but that process was hardly an accident. And there was nothing random about the way every living creature in the world operated. If it was, trees would grow sideways and polar bears would come in assorted colors!

Far from being random, the world around us is very orderly and predictable. Each living organism, from the human being to the smallest amoeba, is created with the knowledge of what it must do to survive and thrive. Unfortunately, imperfections in the structure of the physical entity might make it impossible to do this, but the knowledge is there.

Take, for instance, our own bodies. When we're born, we do not have the learned knowledge of how to breathe, make our hearts beat, or digest food. But our bodies know how to do all these things and millions of other things which are part of living. Even as we get older, our bodies use their own innate intelligence to function as well as the physical structure will allow.

When you cut your finger, you don't intellectually know how to make your blood clot or how to send extra white blood cells to the area to automatically fight infection. You wouldn't be able to "command" your body to form a scab to protect the cut area, or to grow new skin cells over the damaged spot. But your body knows how to do these things.

Your body also knows how to adapt when you are exposed to germs and viruses, eat a spoiled piece of food or strain your back lifting a heavy object. Whether it will be able to react the way it should depends on the state of your physical body.

Because of genetic and environmental factors, the bodies we are born with are not always in perfect condition. In addition, the way we treat our bodies — our diet, lifestyle, and emotional and mental attitudes — have a tremendous affect on our physical condition. If a body is limited by either inherent or acquired weaknesses, innate intelligence alone will not be able to achieve perfect health. But it will always keep trying and working to go in that direction.

Perhaps the most important component, often overlooked even by popular alternative M.D.s, is spinal nerve interference, and this is where chiropractic comes in.

The body's nerve system is an incredibly complex communication network which links the brain to all parts of the body, chemically influencing even the smallest cells. There are miles of nerve fiber running throughout our bodies. No one has been able to count the number of nerve cells in the human body, but it is estimated that there are at least 10-12 billion of them — possibly many, many more.

Over this nerve network, the brain receives constantly updated information from the cells, organs and tissues and instantaneously relays instructions back. The whole process is so fast that scientists have only recently begun to measure the speed of the impulses — and no one has come up with a definitive speed. But you can get an idea of the incredible speed by remembering what happened the last time you grabbed hold of the handle of a hot pot on the stove.

Before you even realized what had happened, you jerked your hand away — and immediately, a blister started forming as a protective response to the injury. You hardly had a chance to yelp in pain, but the cells in your finger had already transmitted the information about the injury to your brain, which responded by instructing other cells to react in a specific way determined by your innate intelligence.

That's exactly what happens with every other cell in your body, all the time. You don't have to burn yourself to trigger the communication system. The flow of information to and from your body is a constant background function which keeps your body as healthy as it can be, given its specific physical limitations.

But what if something interferes with that communication system? What if there is "line noise" as they call it in telephone circuits? What if the messages to and from the brain become even the slightest bit garbled?

The result can range from a slightly less-than-perfect response of a particular tissue cell, to a steadily worsening malfunction of a vital organ or life support system. Either way, your body is not going to be able to do what its innate intelligence knows it has to do to keep optimum health.

The spine is made up of 24 small bones called vertebrae: 7 in the neck, 12 in the mid back, and 5 in the lower back. Most of these vertebrae are shaped somewhat like donuts, with a hole in the middle. The spinal cord fits into and is protected by these ring-shaped bones. Two additional vertebrae at the bottom of the spine, the sacrum and the coccyx, complete what is called the spinal column.

Naturally, nerve endings have to be able to branch out throughout the whole body, so the spinal column isn't merely a solid bone encasing it. Instead, it is a marvel of engineering design! One part is a solid bone which helps bear the weight of our body and head.

The bones stack together in a precise way which allows a "canal" between them, aptly called the "neural canal." It is through this small canal that the primary nerve bundles branch off the spinal cord and make their way to all parts of the body.

If we didn't have to bend, those bones could have been locked into place. But the spine has to be flexible, so its design incorporates a thick, fibrous cushion of cartilage, called an intervertebral disk, that acts as a shock absorber, in the joint between each pair of vertebrae. This allows us to bend, turn, flex and move with relative freedom.

Unfortunately, this need for flexibility means that the size of the canals can be made larger or smaller by movement. Think of it as a door. When the door is open all the way, you can put your hand between it and the wall, near the hinges. But if you accidentally close that door when your hand is there, watch out! If you close it only a little bit, or quickly open it again, you may escape serious damage.

But what if you don't re-open the door right away? What if you close the door on your hand and leave it closed? Before long, even if you haven't shut the door all the way — just enough to "pinch" your fingers — you'll not only be in a great deal of pain, but you'll probably have permanently damaged your hand.

Your nerves pass through the opening in the "doorway" between the vertebrae. Usually, we manage to move freely without ever closing the doorway on these nerves. But sometimes, our vertebrae become misaligned and the door shuts too far. Maybe not all the way ... just enough to create abnormal pressure — enough to make a difference to the flow of nerve impulses through that nerve fiber. The longer the door is left partially closed, the worse the damage will be.

When vertebrae become stuck in an abnormal position, it's called a vertebral subluxation. To be more precise, the subluxation is not merely the presence of a misaligned bone. It also involves the presence of a "neurological insult" to use a technical term. In other words, the misalignment is causing a change in the flow of normal nerve impulses. The nerve "short circuits" and is being disrupted in some way because of the misaligned bones.

The effects of vertebral subluxation on health have been well-documented in the millions of case studies recorded by practicing doctors of chiropractic. It is the chiropractor's job to determine whether there are any subluxations, and introduce the precise amount of force (called an adjustment) to gently — but firmly — unlock the vertebrae and allow them to return to their proper alignment.

This is the single purpose for which the profession of chiropractic was founded, and it remains — after more than a century — the primary goal of traditional, subluxation-centered doctors of chiropractic.

20

Of course, there are other things that can interfere with the proper flow of nerve impulses. Among these are chemicals such as those found in certain foods and drinks, pollutants, and even prescription and over-the-counter drugs. In fact, early chiropractors were the first "body ecologists" to sound an alarm about the damage which could be done by the unwise use of medications, dumped into the most important stream in the world — the human blood stream.

They taught that people can't expect to take a magic pill to improve the function of the bodies. D.D. Palmer expressed this with the phrase, "Above, down, inside, out." He meant that true health comes from within — not from without.

Obviously, this didn't sit well with the evolving medical establishment, which was coming to rely more and more heavily on drugs and surgery to "treat" patients. Doctors began focusing all their attention on so-called scientific breakthroughs — from antibiotics to iron lungs.

It seemed some new drug or device was constantly being brought into the medical arena and the business of modern medicine was born. Fewer and fewer doctors were content being "general family practitioners."

Instead, they wanted to be cardiologists and endocrinologists — to work with a piece of the human body rather than to see the body as a whole, integrated unit.

For these upstart chiropractors to tell patients they had the power within themselves to heal and become healthy was an outrage. Patients needed medical doctors to give them drugs, more hospitals to operate on their organs, deliver their babies, and scientifically treat their diseases. Chiropractors were "quacks" to be avoided at all cost.

By the middle of the 20th century, the medical profession was working hard to bring everyone into the medical model of sickness and disease care. Today, the medical, hospital and drug industries pump billions of dollars into advertising and marketing, and even political manipulation in order to keep the public convinced that the allopathic medical model is the only viable system.

Chapter 3

WHY PEOPLE ARE CONFUSED

The definition of chiropractic is simple: a health care field dedicated to the detection and correction of vertebral subluxation in order to eliminate spinal nerve interference which can adversely affect health. To this, we can add the facts that chiropractic is drug-free, non-invasive and respectful of the body's own innate striving for health. That's it. Clean, simple, and powerful.

Despite its simplicity, the federal government found it necessary to tackle the problem of defining the terms "primary health care provider" as it relates to chiropractic.

In a 1975 letter to the vice-president of Sherman College of Chiropractic, David A. Kindig, M.D., deputy director of the Department of Health, Education and Welfare, had hesitated to define chiropractic. "The responsibility for defining and limiting the scope of practice of any health profession lies in the individual states which, through practice acts and licensure, regulate what it is that independent practitioners may or may not do within that state," he noted. "No federal laws or regulations supersede these."

However, the federal government's involvement with national health care programs such as Medicare and Medicaid forced the agency to examine chiropractic closely and develop a working description so that government personnel, and the public, would understand the terms used in government documents.

Dr. Kindig stated that chiropractors are primary health care providers. Unfortunately, some people, in a desire to practice medicine, insisted this meant they must be able to diagnose and treat the same range of diseases as their medical counterparts.

Yet, Dr. Kindig clearly rejected that notion, saying, "this term does not mandate chiropractors to perform diagnostic examinations of the entire body."

Why, then, is there so much confusion about what chiropractic is and what chiropractors do? If you ask 10 people, you'll get 10 answers. One will say doctors of chiropractic are the ones who "crack backs." Another will say they relieve back pain. A third will claim they cure allergies or headaches. The variations are endless! Only a few will even mention subluxations.

There are several reasons for this confusion.

❖ ❖ ❖

WELL MEANING PATIENTS CAUSE CONFUSION

First, there are all those testimonials from satisfied patients. Of course, chiropractors love to hear from patients who are feeling healthier and happier because of regular chiropractic care. But, as we mentioned before, some patients forget to tell the most important part of the story — that correcting vertebral subluxations allows the intelligence that made the body to heal the body. In their enthusiasm, they give credit to their chiropractor for their "cures."

When a patient tells a friend that her child's ear infections were "cured" by chiropractic, the friend is bound to get the impression that the doctor of chiropractic diagnosed the child's condition and specifically treated it. The same thing goes when a patient tells a co-worker that his migraines disappeared after only a few adjustments. The co-worker will go home thinking chiropractic is a treatment for headaches.

When the friend and the co-worker go to see a chiropractor themselves, they're going to be expecting their doctor to diagnose their illnesses and treat them. When they're told that the purpose of chiropractic is to determine whether they have subluxations in their spine, and correct them, they're bound to be confused.

The way to avoid this confusion and the frustration it can cause is for the doctor to make sure proper educational material is available to patients. On their part, the patients have to play an active role in their own health care and take time to learn about and understand chiropractic.

This isn't as easy as it sounds.

For decades, we've been made to be spectators when it comes to health. We sit back and put our health into the hands of the medical profession. Studies have shown that the vast majority of patients who go to a medical doctor never ask a single question about the doctor's diagnosis or treatment plan!

They never ask about the drugs they are given or even about potential side effects they may experience. Most are too intimidated to demand a second opinion — even in the case of a diagnosis of serious illness.

Often, this is because the attitude of doctors make it clear that they do not have the time or inclination to discuss things with their patients.

They rush them through the examination and out to the receptionist who takes their money or insurance plan information. If a patient does ask a question, the doctor is often patronizing or irritated. That's why so many patients go home and write to their local newspaper's medical columnist.

Almost all questions submitted to these columnists start with the phrase, "I just got back from my doctor's office and I don't understand ..."

This is particularly true for women patients, who are often treated with little respect by medical professionals. The famed "People's Doctor," Robert Mendelsohn, M.D., exposed the blatant sexism within the medical profession in his book, "MalePractice: How Doctors Manipulate Women."

He noted that, "Male chauvinism pervades American medicine from the doors of medical school to the slabs of the hospital morgue." Although this was written in 1982, little has changed since then.

A report published on Nov. 21, 1996 by the Center for Cardiovascular Education found that nearly two-thirds of the nation's primary care doctors didn't realize there were differences between the symptoms of heart disease in women compared to men.

Only 39% of them had medical training in diagnosing heart disease in women, compared to 69% who had been taught how to spot it in male patients.

There are many other similar studies showing that the male-dominated medical profession doesn't take women patients as seriously as they do their male counterparts — which means they don't take the time to explain things.

Particularly when it comes to health, this attitude toward the medical profession is just plain dangerous! Everyone needs to read, ask questions, and make the effort to learn.

That applies to chiropractic as well. If you don't take the time to understand what chiropractic can do for you, you're not going to get as much out of it as those individuals who are well-informed. And, you risk the dissatisfaction that comes with misunderstanding.

> **Be not alarmed as to great truth. It may be obscured for a time by error, but always to rise in greater glory.**
>
> **— B.J. Palmer**

DELIBERATELY MISLEADING THE PUBLIC

The second reason for all the confusion about chiropractic is, once more, the medical profession. As noted in the previous chapter, medical doctors were at first curious about — then afraid of — this new health care field. If people adopted it as their primary approach to health, there would be far less need for medical doctors and their drugs, surgery and therapies.

Because the field was so new, there was no such thing as a chiropractic license. Medical doctors, who had to pass tests to get their licenses to practice, were angry about losing patients to people who were, in their eyes, "laymen." To stop this exodus of patients, medical doctors tried to put their chiropractic competitors out of business by accusing them of practicing medicine without a license. Because they enjoyed relatively high status in our society, they were able to convince legislators and law enforcement officials that chiropractors were offering medical treatment.

D.D. Palmer was arrested in 1906 and was the first to serve a jail sentence for practicing medicine without a license.

"I am here for a principle which is chiropractic," he stated in May of that year. "This is mine. I discovered and developed it. No medical school has ever practiced or used it. In doing so, I am not practicing surgery, medicine, or obstetrics. I am opposed to the practice of medicine in all its branches."

D.D. Palmer continued, "After I went to jail, several parties phoned my home and others offered to lend me money with which to pay my fine. I am not in a cell for lack of princi**pal** but for an abundance of princi**ple**."

Other chiropractors were dragged into court as well, and many ended up serving time in jail. In Jan. 1923, chiropractors B.F. Lear and W.E. Quartier were sentenced to pay either a $500 fine or spend 833 days in jail, the maximum sentence for a first offense. They both chose the Trumbull County Jail in Warren, Ohio.

Conditions in the jails were difficult for these doctors, who had lived quiet, peaceful lives before they became the target of the medical witchhunt. Yet, most managed to maintain their courage and their spirits.

W.D. Adrian of McConnelsville, in the Morgan County Jail for 500 days, wrote, "We see an occasional rat but all the bugs apparently were killed last summer in a big raid on the jail. I could stand some springs or a mattress on the bars I sleep on. But outside of this and the disagreeable dispositions of some of the prisoners, I am getting along nicely."

For others, their resentment of the medical establishment was mixed with a strong sense of determination.

In a letter written from jail to B.J. Palmer —D.D. Palmer's son who had taken up his father's leadership of the fledgling profession — Harriet Clemens mused, "We have been guests of the AMA for 72 days and have not worn out our welcome yet. Great isn't it? They still feed us and give us a place to sleep so why should we worry? No doubt you have heard of us getting our release providing we would quit practicing. They must think we are easy; we could have done that before we came down here."

For some, though, the experience took a terrible toll. According to a news report at the time of his death, Dr. Albert Ivnick, a chiropractor from Cleveland, Ohio "never recovered from the effects of exposure at Warrensville Workhouse, and has been in bed from time to time since resuming his practice in February, and finally passed away last night. He leaves a wife and four children." He, too, had been imprisoned for helping people live healthier lives through chiropractic.

Despite the conditions and the harassment, chiropractors never gave up the fight. Many even continued a practice of sorts in jail. One wrote: "This is our 36th day and all are strongly preaching the gospel of chiropractic... we are adjusting some of the prisoners in jail. Sometimes we have to use the TM and break as we have to reach through the bars, but we do the work just the same."

And when they were released, they refused to bow to the pressure, returning to their practices and their grateful patients. W.C. Swaggard of Millersburg, Ohio, wrote to B.J. Palmer saying, "I was dismissed from jail at 5 p.m. and at 7 p.m. was adjusting patients at the office, and have been going right along since, the same as I

> **To compromise with anything medical in legislation, is to accept something short of full freedom, which would be part of slavery.** — B.J. Palmer

was before I was arrested."

Through it all, chiropractors kept practicing chiropractic and continued to attract new patients who heard about them through "word of mouth." They tried to explain that they weren't practicing "medicine" at all. Far from it! They kept pointing out that medicine deals with the diagnosis and treatment of illness and disease — chiropractic deals with correcting vertebral subluxations and health.

But the medical doctors and their supporters were far more powerful than the small but growing number of chiropractors and their patients. They kept insisting that chiropractors were "practicing medicine without a license" and demanding that they be arrested or at least prohibited from practicing.

✻ ✻ ✻

CREDITED WITH CURES

While the lawmakers listened, the general public didn't. More and more people began going to chiropractors, particularly when medical treatments didn't help them. Incredible "success" stories started circulating from satisfied patients. "It cured my arthritis," one would say. "I had been crippled for 20 years, and now I can walk." Another would tell the story about a baby who had colic and had been taking medications for months — but was "cured" by a few chiropractic adjustments. Some said their sight or hearing was restored by chiropractic. Others claimed it stopped their migraines or cleared up their allergies.

Chiropractors found it necessary to keep emphasizing that these "miraculous" cures were the direct result of unleashing the patient's own natural healing power from within.

Unlike their medical counterparts, who seemed eager to

snatch the credit for any improvement in a patient's health, chiropractors made sure people knew that the adjustment corrected the subluxations — the person's own innate wisdom did the rest. If anyone was practicing medicine without a license, it was the patients themselves — and they were doing a very good job of it!

Within just a few years, the profession started growing too quickly for it to be completely destroyed. In 1907, in a court case in Wisconsin, a chiropractor was found innocent of the charge of practicing medicine without a license. In the landmark decision, the judge and jury agreed that he wasn't practicing medicine, but an entirely different form of health care: chiropractic.

Over the next two decades, state after state began passing legislation specifically geared to making chiropractic a licensed health care field. Chiropractors now had their own non-medical category, and the medical doctors could no longer have them thrown into jail.

Once chiropractors were allowed to legally open up practices, their patient volume increased significantly — and so did the testimonials from patients. Despite attempts by their doctors to educate them, chiropractic patients often failed to grasp the truth about correcting subluxations and how their lives were improved from Above-Down-Inside-Out.

Instead, they understandably were more concerned with the fact that they were feeling healthier than ever before. So, they told their friends and neighbors their "miracle cures" came from the hands of their chiropractors.

That made the medical establishment more furious and frightened than ever before. The profession was facing what could be a true competitor, one which could possibly knock medicine off its throne as the dominant health care system in America. M.D.s weren't going to go down in defeat without a battle.

As it turns out, medicine chose to go to war with chiropractic.

The first attack was to embark on a campaign of misinformation in order to confuse and deceive the public. They completely ignored the teachings of the Palmers and misrepresented chiropractic as a "medical" field which used unscientific, unproven, and potentially dangerous methods. At the same time, they tried to debunk it as a hoax — although this was more difficult since so many people were telling their own true-life stories about their renewed health, improved function, and greater quality of life.

❖ ❖ ❖

TAKING IT TO COURT

The American Medical Association (AMA) spent millions of dollars in an attempt to destroy chiropractic. The AMA is a professional trade association whose purpose is to protect the business interests of medical doctors. Presently, fewer than half of all M.D.s actually belong to this group, yet it still wields a lot of power.

For years, the AMA released a barrage of misinformation to the public and to its own members. It even forbid its member doctors from associating with or referring patients to chiropractors. Having anything to do with chiropractors was considered unethical and unprofessional. They publicly ridiculed the concept of subluxations and refused to support any scientific research which

> ## It is impossible to be right when the reason for action is wrong.
>
> ### — B.J. Palmer

would help prove that chiropractic had value.

Unfortunately, many people were scared off by this campaign, and an entire generation of patients and medical doctors were brainwashed into believing that chiropractic was merely "unscientific quackery."

Finally, in 1976, a group of chiropractors decided to fight back. They filed a lawsuit against the AMA and other medical associations which were involved in the mis-information campaign. They spent years gathering evidence to prove their contention that the medical community had engaged in a deliberate attempt to eliminate competition by maligning chiropractic.

The AMA claimed it was merely acting in the best interest of patients, since chiropractic was not only ineffective but dangerous. However, the chiropractors brought in their own evidence — which showed just the opposite.

In the end, the chiropractors won, and the AMA and its co-defendants were found guilty of a conspiracy to create a medical monopoly. On August 27, 1987, U.S. District Court Judge Susan Getzendanner issued her opinion that, as far back as 1963, the AMA had been working aggressively both "overtly and covertly" to eliminate the profession of chiropractic. She issued a permanent court injunction against the AMA to prevent such behavior in the future.

Although the AMA complied with the letter of the injunction, many feel they never complied with its spirit. There is still a very strong anti-chiropractic feeling among the organization and many practicing medical doctors.

In recent years, the medical profession has been carrying on another campaign. They finally realized they can't destroy chiropractic — but they are still hoping to limit it.

The medical community today tries to paint a picture of chiropractic as a last resort "treatment" for low back pain in adults. It steadfastly refuses to discuss the validity of subluxation correction (although many medical doctors are quietly trying to learn "spinal manipulative therapy" for their own practices) and criticizes the use of chiropractic for children or for patients who have no symptoms but simply want to be healthier and live a wellness lifestyle. Medical authorities always make sure the media includes misguided "warnings" when chiropractic is mentioned!

Again, as in the early days of the profession, it hasn't stopped patients from going to chiropractors. More than 25 million people visit their chiropractors each year, and it is being introduced into nations around the world.

But, the continued assault on chiropractic did a great deal of damage. After decades of hearing lies and distortions about the profession, most people have still never heard the word "subluxation" unless it is in a derogatory way in material put out by the medical establishment and they have seldom been exposed to the fact that their own bodies have an innate ability to heal.

* * *

CONFUSION AMONG D.C.S THEMSELVES

After a century of being misrepresented, it's not surprising

> ## Who can anchor to an unanchored mind?
>
> — B.J. Palmer

that chiropractic is misunderstood by the general public. It's harder to understand, however, why there appears to be confusion or disagreement within the profession itself. There are various groups within chiropractic who disagree completely with the traditional definition of chiropractic, who are actively trying to redefine the discipline — and who often make things even more confusing for the public.

Ever since the early days of D.D. and B.J. Palmer, some chiropractors felt their role went beyond the detection and correction of subluxations. They made broad (and at times unsubstantiated) claims that chiropractic could "cure" any number of diseases and ailments. They saw vertebral subluxations as the cause of diseases and, by correcting the spinal misalignments, felt they were treating the diseases themselves.

In doing so, they definitely were treading on the toes of the medical doctors, since their purpose was to treat the result of subluxations rather than to correct the subluxation itself. This is a very subtle difference, but an important one. Even though they might have conducted the same examinations and given the same adjustments, the fact that their objective was the diagnosis and treatment of diseases and physical conditions caused them to step over the line separating chiropractic from medicine.

Later, as the attack on chiropractic by medicine intensified, there was an added reason on the part of these chiropractors to try to appear more "medical." Many of them felt they would be safe from attack if they imitated medical doctors. They tried to distance themselves from the "disreputable" chiropractic profession by disowning much of what made chiropractic unique. They adopted the medical objective of diagnosing and treating diseases, used medical terminology instead of chiropractic language, and even went so far as to wear white lab coats and drape stethoscopes around their necks.

35

To many, it seemed as though they truly wanted to be medical doctors! Even today, many doctors of chiropractic prefer to be called chiropractic physicians, or doctors of chiropractic medicine — terms which are not in favor with the profession as a whole. Some chiropractors have even fought to change their state's licensing laws to permit D.C.s to write drug prescriptions and perform minor surgeries!

The differences in the way individual chiropractors think about chiropractic and what they hold as their practice objective has led to the development of a classification system to categorize risk. This system was first devised by Chiropractic Benefit Services (CBS) for its professional liability program. CBS realized that the differences in the way doctors practice was reflected in their relative risk when being sued for malpractice. The more "medical" the practice, the greater the chance of being sued. Those doctors who maintain a traditional or subluxation-based practice are the least likely to be taken to court.

According to the CBS classifications, there are four types of doctors:

CLASS 1:

Doctors of chiropractic in Class 1 have as their sole practice objective the detection and correction of the vertebral subluxation. While they may be aware of a patient's symptoms or specific health problems, they do not attempt to treat those symptoms or conditions.

In addition, they use an informed consent document (such as the "Terms of Acceptance") which clearly explains their practice objective. In their Report of Unusual Findings, they note findings they observed not related to vertebral subluxations, but they do not attempt to diagnose those findings, make specific recommendations, or referrals. They accept the responsibility of informing their patients of the unusual finding, allowing them to determine the need for medical advice or care.

Class 1 chiropractors use manual adjusting techniques, which can include hand-held devices such as the Atlas Orthogonal Instrument, Integrator or Activator, etc.

In addition, they may use traction, extremity adjusting, massage, hot and cold packs, orthotics, or other non-invasive modalities which they consider necessary in order to properly correct subluxations, or which they feel will help patients hold their adjustments.

Nutritional supplements, and exercise or lifestyle counseling may be included if it is specifically for the purpose of helping the patient to live a subluxation-free life.

Class 1 doctors do not use therapeutic agents, including nutritional supplements, homeopathic or naturopathic remedies, to treat diseases or suppress symptoms.

Surface electromyography (SEMG) in the paraspinal area may be used to measure a variety of physiological changes to determine if subluxation exists. Evidence-based documentation from spinal range-of-motion and computerized muscle testing studies fall within Class 1. Skin temperature measurement instruments may be used to evaluate neurological changes associated with vertebral subluxation.

No diagnostic or treatment modalities should be used which are not directly related to the detection and correction of vertebral subluxation. X-ray and other imaging techniques may be used to assist in determining the presence of vertebral subluxation in the spine.

Approximately 35% of the profession falls into this category, this would include doctors of straight chiropractic who may refer to themselves as subluxation-*centered*. These doctors believe that since their sole objective is the correction of vertebral subluxation their sole intervention is the adjustment to correct vertebral subluxation. This category would also include other subluxation-based chiropractors who see the adjustment as the foundation of what they do, but add additional procedures to their care.

CLASS 2:

Doctors of chiropractic in Class 2 focus on the detection and correction of the vertebral subluxation. In addition, they may address neuromusculoskeletal complaints and treat spinal-related conditions and symptoms such as strains and sprains.

To achieve their practice objective, doctors in Class 2 may utilize everything included under Class 1, and, modalities such as electrical stimulation, ultrasound, diathermy, whirlpool, cryotherapy, orthopedic supports, homeopathy related to the spine, athletic taping, etc. — all for the purpose of detecting or correcting vertebral subluxation or diagnosing and treating neuromusculoskeletal complaints.

Although invasive procedures are not used, neurologic and orthopedic tests are sometimes performed.

D.C.s who are also Certified Chiropractic Sports Physicians may qualify for this Class if they do not treat disease processes or use any modality other than those we've described.

An estimated 50% of the profession falls into this category.

CLASS 3:

Doctors of chiropractic are considered to be in Class 3 if their practice objective is full body diagnosis and treatment of disease, and they use any modality allowed within the scope of chiropractic licensure with the exception of gynecology, minor surgery or manipulation under anesthesia.

These doctors incorporate spinal manipulative therapy (SMT) or other therapeutic tools. They attempt to diagnose an unlimited number of conditions such as diabetes, kidney disease, heart disease, cancer, multiple sclerosis, etc. Class 3 doctors treat their patients' disease or their related symptoms directly.

They perform full-body diagnosis using medical techniques such as diagnostic blood work, urinalysis, full-body X-ray, etc.

To treat patient health problems, they may use a variety of tools including galvanic stimulation, nutritional counseling, homeopathy, fasting, acupuncture or meridian therapy, colon irrigation and many other techniques. Doctors offering acupuncture must comply with OSHA Guidelines for use of disposable needles.

Either implicitly or explicitly, Class 3 doctors shape patient expectation to include medical diagnosis of non-chiropractic conditions, and doctors are expected to make such diagnoses correctly and/or refer patients to appropriate health care professionals.

The Class 3 category specifically excludes gynecological procedures, minor surgery (including casting of fractures), or manipulation under anesthesia.

An estimated 10% of all chiropractors can be categorized as Class 3 D.C.s

CLASS 4:

Sharing the same general practice objective as Class 3 doctors, Class 4 doctors diagnose and treat medical conditions and diseases within the chiropractic scope of practice for their state. This may include but is not limited to gynecological exams, minor surgery or manipulation under anesthesia.

In addition to all of the diagnostic and treatment modalities included in Class 3, Class 4 doctors might perform gynecological and breast exams, minor surgery, cast fractures, give manipulation under anesthesia, prescribe drugs and vitamin injections, perform acupuncture, use MRI/CT scans for medical diagnostic purposes, use invasive electromyography, and conduct other medical procedures allowed by law.

Doctors who hold diplomate degrees and present themselves as specialists or who receive referrals from other chiropractors on the basis of their specialized training or certification are considered Class 4 chiropractors. This includes doctors with any of the following Diplomate credentials: American Chiropractic Board of Nutrition, American Board of Chiropractic Orthopedists, American Chiropractic Board of Radiology, American Board of Chiropractic Internists, American Chiropractic Board of Rehabilitation, Chiropractic Academy of Neurology and American Chiropractic Board of Occupational Health.

On insurance claims, Class 4 doctors list a wide variety of medical codes both for diagnostic and treatment purposes.

An estimated 5% of all chiropractors can be categorized as Class 4.

As this description of the risk classification system plainly shows, it's no wonder patients, the general public and even some chiropractors themselves are not at all sure what chiropractic is about!

Chapter 4

IS THE SUBLUXATION IMPORTANT?

W hen medical doctors criticize chiropractic, they often claim that there really is no such thing as a subluxation. Yet, the concept of subluxation is not new, and even ancient healers apparently used crude spinal adjustments in an attempt to correct nerve flow.

Their understanding of the flow of energy throughout the body was called "vitalism," and there is ample written evidence that many cultures incorporated spinal manipulation into their health care. In fact, the job of the traditional "bone setter" was not only to set broken bones, but to straighten misaligned bones in the spine and other areas of the skeleton.

But it wasn't until D.D. Palmer began to study the relationship between vertebral misalignments and health closely that the concept was fully recognized. His use of specific adjustments on individual vertebra made his technique unique and started the entire profession which is now the second largest primary health care field in the world.

Unfortunately — partly because of the tremendous opposition it faced from the medical profession — chiropractic research lagged behind for many years. Foundations willing to pump millions of dollars into research to develop new drugs, which could then produce billions of dollars in revenue, weren't willing to fund chiropractic research that might prove the drugs weren't needed.

The Association of Chiropractic Colleges (ACC) is a group consisting of all chiropractic college presidents in North America. It defines the subluxation as a "complex of functional and/or structural and/or pathological articular changes that compromise neural integrity and may influence organ system function and general health."

The ACC states its position on chiropractic this way:

Chiropractic is a health care discipline which emphasizes the inherent recuperative power of the body to heal itself without the use of drugs or surgery.

The practice of chiropractic focuses on the relationship between structure (primarily the spine) and function (as coordinated by the nervous system) and how that relationship affects the preservation and restoration of health. In addition, Doctors of Chiropractic recognize the value and responsibility of working in cooperation with other health care practitioners when in the best interest of the patient.

> **Common sense gives power to knowledge and makes wisdom in the process.**
>
> — B.J. Palmer

The Association of Chiropractic Colleges continues to foster a unique, distinct chiropractic profession that serves as a health care discipline for all. The ACC advocates a profession that generates, develops and utilizes the highest level of evidence possible in the provision of effective, prudent, and cost-conscious patient evaluation and care.

Individual colleges agree about the importance of subluxation correction.

In a survey of chiropractic colleges in the U.S. and Canada, taken by *The Chiropractic Journal* in Oct. 1993, here's what some of them had to say:

Cleveland Chiropractic College and Cleveland Chiropractic College-Los Angeles: "The central element in Cleveland Colleges' approach to chiropractic education and practice is the focus on the relationship between movement or position of spinal vertebrae and the nervous system, and the effect of this relationship on the restoration and maintenance of health and wellness."

The Palmer University System: "(Our college) embraces the philosophy that life is intelligent; the human body possesses inherent potential to maintain itself in a natural state of homeostasis through its innate/inborn intelligence ... maintains that the science of chiropractic emphasizes the relationship between structure, primarily of the spinal column and the nervous system, and how that relationship affects function and health. Implicit within this statement is the significance of the nervous system to health and the effect of the subluxation complex upon the nervous system..."

Sid E. Williams, B.S., D.C., President and Founder of Life University: "Those who treat the WHOLE body must have earned educational credentials which can only be achieved through a curriculum sharply different from chiropractic in scope, orientation and application. Academic standards established by state law and

43

CCE regulations are fully adequate to qualify the current chiropractic practitioner <u>provided</u> he limit his scope of practice to that provided for by state law. He must recognize that chiropractic as a profession has a mandate for only a limited scope of practice provided for by his education and qualifications.

Expanding chiropractic practices and procedures beyond this limited scope will result in exposing the entire profession to valid criticism that we lack the education and training to engage in a large scope of practice, especially whole body treatment.

In sum, chiropractic embodies a unique philosophy based on the Innate, the vertebral subluxation and the specific chiropractic adjustment. The ideas these words describe unite to make chiropractic a coherent health system."

Sherman College of Straight Chiropractic: "We teach that contributing to health through the safe correction of subluxation is the only reason for (chiropractic) practice. We teach that the innate wisdom of the body is always striving to correct any abnormal condition within the body and that subluxation disturbs nerve function and modifies mental impulses; thereby diminishing the body's innate striving to regain and maintain its own health."

Another explanation for the importance of the vertebral subluxation was given by Dr. Christopher Kent, president of the Council on Chiropractic Practice, who was named "Chiropractic Researcher of the Year" in 1991 by the International Chiropractors Association and in 1994 by The World Chiropractic Alliance.

"Vertebral subluxation represents the heart and soul of chiropractic. It is our raison d'etre as a profession," he said in an article in *The Chiropractic Journal*. "Health is dependent upon maintaining appropriate tone in the nervous system. . . The ability to maintain tone requires a nervous system free of interference. Restoration of tone is dependent upon correction of vertebral subluxations."

Chapter 5

THE CHIROPRACTIC EXAMINATION FOR VERTEBRAL SUBLUXATION

(AKA SPINAL NERVE INTERFERENCE)

To find out what chiropractic is really all about, and what a patient should expect when going to a chiropractor, let's first take a look at the Guideline developed by the Council on Chiropractic Practice (CCP).

The CCP was formed in July 1995 and is made up of an inter-disciplinary team of distinguished chiropractors, medical physicians, research scientists, attorneys, and consumer representatives.

> ### Where there is no vision the people perish.
>
> ### — B.J. Palmer

In recent years, especially when health care reform was a hot issue in Washington, the federal government has insisted that each health care discipline develop guidelines for their practitioners — or the government would do it for them! Since it was obvious that government health officials (made up mostly of medical doctors) wouldn't understand subluxation-based chiropractic, the chiropractic profession decided to work to develop an acceptable set of guidelines which all practitioners could use.

The stated mission of the CCP is "to develop evidence-based guidelines, conduct research and perform other functions that will enhance the practice of chiropractic for the benefit of the consumer."

The CCP developed these practice guidelines with the active participation of practicing doctors, consultants, seminar leaders, and technique experts. A group of experts, chosen for their special skills and experience, directed a review of numerous studies and other evidence. In the end, they came up with the first set of evidence-based guidelines which could be used by doctors, insurance companies, government health care officials — and the public.

The Guidelines were developed to protect the ability of fami-

> **We never know how far reaching something we may think, say or do today will affect the lives of millions tomorrow.**
>
> **— B.J. Palmer**

lies to obtain subluxation-based wellness care, including patients who weren't displaying any particular symptoms, but just wanted to remain as healthy as possible.

The document is set up in sections, with separate chapters covering every aspect of chiropractic care from the initial examination to the final disposition of a case. Although it can be very technical, the basic information gives a clear picture of what chiropractic is really all about.

To understand the Guidelines and what they mean to patients, we're going to take you through the entire process, from the time the patient first visits a chiropractor.

To begin with, the Guidelines state that the initial chiropractic examination should begin with a thorough case history, which involves getting general information from the patient. This information often includes finding out why the person has come to the doctor in the first place, as well as what symptoms or conditions may be present. Of course, other personal history such as family history, past health history, occupation, etc. may also be included.

If you recall, we explained earlier that chiropractic is NOT concerned directly with symptoms and diseases. It may seem strange, then, that the case history includes questions about health history and the presence of symptoms. It's important to realize that, as the Guidelines point out, "The purpose of the case history is to elicit information which might reveal salient points concerning the patient's spinal and general health that may lead the chiropractor to elect appropriate examination procedures."

In other words, chiropractors aren't trying to find out whether or not the patient has a chronic allergy problem in order to diagnose or treat that problem, but to gather clues as to specific areas of the spine which may be subluxated. Doctors can decide on the best examination procedure to use once they have all the related information.

47

THE PHYSICAL EXAMINATION

The chiropractic exam itself can include a number of different tests. Most chiropractors will begin by taking one or more X-rays since it has been proven to be one of the most effective tools for detecting the misalignments which may signal vertebral subluxations. The CCP Guidelines noted that "Imaging is a necessary component of a number of different chiropractic analyses. The preponderance of evidence supports the reliability of these procedures when properly performed."

The chiropractor is particularly well trained in taking and reading X-rays. In fact, a review of the curriculum for both medical and chiropractic students showed that the average medical student was required to take only 148 hours of radiology — but the chiropractic student was given 360 hours of study in this critical subject!

In addition to X-rays, many chiropractors are using other imaging techniques, including videofluoroscopy, which is somewhat like an X-ray movie picture. It may be used when the doctor wishes to check for abnormal motion patterns.

Other more complex imaging systems, such as Magnetic Resonance Imaging (MRI), Computed Tomography (CT), Spinal Ultrasonography, and Radioisotope Scanning may even be used in unusual cases.

But, since the vertebral subluxation is more than the actual misalignment of the bone, the doctor of chiropractic has to do more than take an X-ray. No matter how sophisticated the imaging tests, most chiropractors rely heavily on their own physical examination of the patient's spine, involving some or all of the following:

Range of Motion

One of the main components of the vertebral subluxation is a distortion or impairment of voluntary movement, called "dyskinesia." In patients, this usually means difficulty turning their head or body from side to side, or forward to back. Often, patients will be able to turn to the left a lot further than they can to the right (or vice versa). Some patients come into their chiropractors hardly able to turn their heads at all! Although they may think all they have is a "stiff neck," often it's because they are subluxated.

This impaired range of motion can be tested and measured very accurately. The doctor will have the patient stand and move the body or head side to side, or forward and back. By measuring how far the head or the body can move — how much "range of motion" there is in various parts of the spine — the doctor can get valuable clues as to the presence of vertebral subluxations. There are also sophisticated instruments, like the inclinometer, which can be used to measure this indication of subluxations.

Postural Checks

The way you hold your body can be a good indication of the proper alignment of your spine. The doctor will visually check various "reference points" and note the tilt and balance of each. A patient who stands with one shoulder higher than the other, for example, might have a severe vertebral subluxation which could cause serious health damage.

Leg Length Check

This is one of the more common chiropractic examinations. The patient lies down, and the doctor visually checks and measures the length of each leg. Often only a fraction of an inch discrepancy can signal the presence of a subluxated spine.

Palpation

After years of chiropractic college training and clinical practice, doctors of chiropractic learn to "feel" for subluxations in the spine with the tips of their fingers. Most are remarkably accurate with this type of examination, and can also become aware of any tenderness, soreness or discomfort experienced by the patient as a result of having vertebral subluxations.

Instrumentation

In recent years, chiropractic examinations have become more and more sophisticated, and D.C.s now have quite a few tools at their disposal with which to perform objective tests for vertebral subluxation.

Some tests, like surface electromyography, allow doctors to actually measure the electrical energy expended by the body. This is important since another key component of vertebral subluxation is what is known as "dysponesis," or abnormal involuntary muscle activity. Examination devices which measure skin temperature can help spot abnormalities in the autonomic nervous system (which regulates the action of organs, glands, and blood vessels). This abnormality is called "dysautonomia" and can be another component of the vertebral subluxation.

Other tests can involve computerized muscle strength testing and other related procedures. These may or may not include the use of special instruments or test devices. At no time will a doctor of chiropractic use any invasive procedures to detect subluxations.

> ## No one is useless in the world who lightens the burdens of it for anyone else.
>
> ### — B.J. Palmer

WHAT ARE THEY LOOKING FOR?

As you can see, the examination can include a number of different physical tests as well as the taking of X-rays or other images. What, exactly, is the chiropractor looking for? For one thing and one thing only — evidence of vertebral subluxation.

This is extremely important to understand. The chiropractic tests and examinations are NOT conducted to look for or find any non-chiropractic condition. Patients who have misunderstood the purpose of the chiropractic examination (or who, unfortunately, have been misled by more medically oriented chiropractic physicians) have occasionally accused the doctor of malpractice because later it was discovered they had a medical problem which the D.C. didn't detect. They may later be diagnosed with cancer or diabetes, or an internal injury. They had made an assumption that the chiropractor, having given them such a complete examination, should have noticed those things.

Yet, diagnosing specific diseases or conditions is an extremely

51

complex process. To accurately detect a disease, a physician normally has to be looking specifically for that disease. Few ailments are "discovered" accidentally. That's why a medical doctor checking for an ear infection isn't likely to diagnose a person's heart murmur.

Even when a medical doctor is attempting a full body diagnosis, the accuracy rate is often very low. The high number of "false positives" or missed diagnoses makes it evident that detecting many internal ailments is difficult even when the doctor is looking for them. When the examination is totally geared to detecting evidence of vertebral subluxation — not a specific medical condition or disease — the task becomes almost impossible.

That's why, when chiropractic doctors examine patients for vertebral subluxation, they aren't necessarily going to spot unrelated physical ailments. They may, in the course of their examinations, notice something unusual in the X-ray or the physical tests — something that comes to their attention that, while not typical, isn't an indication of a subluxation. The doctor then will inform the patient that an "unusual finding" was observed. Since, however, it is not within the scope of chiropractic, the chiropractor will not attempt to identify this finding or speculate on its cause or effect.

The greatest thing in the world is where we stand and in what direction we are going.

— B.J. Palmer

To do so would be totally unfair to the patient, who has a right to expect the chiropractor to focus on the area of his or her expertise — the detection and correction of vertebral subluxation. Taking guesses as to the identity of a non-chiropractic finding would be irresponsible.

Since chiropractors normally approach their work as a partnership in health with their patients, they respect the patients' rights and ability to make judgments and decisions about their own health care. The patient, once informed that the doctor has observed a non-chiropractic finding, is free to decide whether or not to go to another health care practitioner to discover the meaning of that finding.

Naturally, in order to achieve optimum health, it is always suggested that non-chiropractic treatment of a medical condition be sought without stopping the chiropractic care. After all, even if a patient decides to obtain medical treatment of a specific disease, his or her body will respond better if its nerve flow is unimpaired.

PUT IT IN WRITING

This difference in a chiropractic examination and a medical examination is so critical that many D.C.s take extra time to explain it to their patients. They do not want patients thinking that the exam will enable the doctor to detect any diseases, conditions or injuries which aren't directly related to the spinal nerve interference. They want to make sure the patient's expectation is based on the real purpose of chiropractic.

Many doctors go one step further. They know that going to ANY health care practitioner for the first time can be stressful. It's usually not as bad when the doctor is a chiropractor, but it can make the person a bit anxious. In addition, the information patients are given on the first visit — from background on chiropractic to details about spinal nerve interference — can be overwhelming! Add to that the fact that many people go to chiropractors when they are sick or in pain. The end result is that, sometimes, patients don't fully absorb what they're being told about the extent and purpose of chiropractic examinations.

To solve this problem, doctors of chiropractic often use an informed consent form which clearly states — in writing — what the doctor will look for during the exam and what he or she will do if any non-chiropractic findings are noted. One popular form is the "Terms of Acceptance" form developed by The World Chiropractic Alliance and used extensively by Chiropractic Benefit Services.

Terms of Acceptance

When a patient seeks chiropractic health care and we accept a patient for such care, it is essential for both to be working towards the same objective.

Chiropractic has only one goal. It is important that each patient understand both the objective and the method that will be used to attain it. This will prevent any confusion or disappointment.

Adjustment: An adjustment is the specific application of forces to facilitate the body's correction of spinal nerve interference. Our chiropractic method of correction is by specific adjustments of the spine.

Health: A state of optimal physical, mental and social well-being, not merely the absence of infirmity.

Vertebral Subluxation: Also known as spinal nerve interference. A misalignment of one or more of the 24 vertebra in the spinal column which causes alteration of nerve function and interference to the transmission of mental impulses, resulting in a lessening of the body's innate ability to express its maximum health potential.

We do not offer to diagnose or treat any disease or condition other than vertebral subluxation. However, if during the course of a chiropractic spinal examination, we encounter non-chiropractic or unusual findings, we will advise you. If you desire advice, diagnosis or treatment for those findings, we will recommend that you seek the services of another health care provider.

Regardless of what the disease is called, we do not offer to treat it. Nor do we offer advice regarding treatment prescribed by others. OUR ONLY PRACTICE OBJECTIVE is to eliminate a major interference to the expression of the body's innate wisdom. Our only method is specific adjusting to correct vertebral subluxations.

I, _____ have read and fully understand the above statements.

All questions regarding the doctor's objectives pertaining to my care in this office have been answered to my complete satisfaction. I therefore accept chiropractic care on this basis.

_____   _____
                (signature)   (date)

Consent to evaluate and adjust a minor child

I, _____ being the parent or legal guardian of _____ have read and fully understand the above terms of acceptance and hereby grant permission for my child to receive chiropractic are.

Pregnancy Release

This is to certify that to the best of my knowledge I am not pregnant and the above doctor and his/her associates have my permission to perform an x-ray evaluation. I have been advised that x-ray can be hazardous to an unborn child. Date of last menstrual period: _____

_____   _____
                (signature)   (date)

55

When doctors notice something unusual which isn't related to the vertebral subluxation, they often use another form so the patient can clearly understand the doctor's verbal explanation. The following form is typical of those used by chiropractic offices around the world:

Report of Unusual Findings

On _____ *(date): my doctor,*
_____, *advised me that unusual non-chiropractic findings were noted in my X-rays or — during my examination during an office visit conversation/consultation — I asked the doctor questions about my symptoms. I now understand that the nature of the problem we discussed is NOT within the scope of chiropractic. The doctor recommended that if I desire advice, diagnosis or treatment for this matter, I should seek the services of an additional health care provider. I understand that seeking advice from another type of health care provider should not interfere with the subluxation correction care currently being provided by this office.*

_____ _____
Patient's Signature *Doctor's Signature*

We rejoice in the power to be a channel for the expression of the divine purpose.

— B.J. Palmer

Chapter 6

CHIROPRACTIC CARE FOR THE SUBLUXATION

Once the chiropractor has finished the examination, and the patient understands completely what can be expected from the care to be given, it's time to correct those subluxations.

Although some patients and doctors refer to their chiropractic care as "treatment," that term is usually considered too medical to apply to chiropractic. After all, D.C.s are not "treating" anything. The word also implies that there is a disease or medical condition which needs to be fixed.

The chiropractor's real job is to restore normal nerve function to the patient by correcting any misalignments discovered during the chiropractic examination. And many patients come in regularly even when they are feeling great, just because they want to stay that way. The concept of treatment doesn't apply at all here.

Instead, chiropractors usually refer to what they offer as "chiropractic care," a phrase which far more accurately reflects their non-medical purpose as well as their sense of compassion for their patients.

Chiropractic care consists primarily of spinal adjustments which are specifically given to correct vertebral subluxation. The CCP definition of an adjustment is "the specific application of force to facilitate the body's correction of vertebral subluxation."

Note that this is NOT the same as the spinal manipulation therapy now offered by some physical therapists and medical doctors. Ask them what the subluxation is, and you're likely to get a blank stare or an angry retort. No other health care professional, other than the chiropractor, applies the specific application of force known as the adjustment for the explicit purpose of correcting vertebral subluxation!

Although all have the same purpose, there are many different styles of chiropractic adjustments, called techniques. All of the commonly used techniques have been well studied and are practiced by many doctors of chiropractic around the country. The choice of technique depends on the individual doctors and the specific cases they're working on.

Many techniques require only the hands — and talents — of the doctor. Some, however, will use hand-held devices such as an Atlas Orthogonal Instrument, Integrator or Activator, etc.

There are a number of other factors involved in how well the adjustment holds, particularly in the case of subluxations which have been present for a long time. The body tends to get used to the position it's in and the muscles around it strengthen or weaken in response to the misalignment. An adjustment will often "unlock" vertebrae from their improper alignment, but it's then up to the body to let the bones settle back into the right position. The body's innate striving for health is strong and it will work hard to get into normal alignment. Even so, sometimes a person's posture, activities, or even physical or emotional stress level will be obstacles in the body's way.

58

> # You can learn anything listening to your Innate.
>
> — B.J. Palmer

HOW LONG DOES CARE LAST?

One of the first questions most patients ask their doctor of chiropractic is, "How many times will I have to come in to see you before I'm healthy?" That's like asking your dentist how many times you'll have to come in before your teeth are "healthy."

Before you can get an answer, you need to figure out what you mean by "healthy."

In the case of your teeth, the short term outlook might interpret "better" to mean whenever you can get through the day without a toothache, or, whenever all your cavities are filled. But what about six months from now? Do you really expect one root canal — which stops the pain you're having at the moment — to make your teeth healthy? Are teeth healthy because you just had three fillings?

The other way to look at healthy teeth is the long-term outlook. After all, you're going to have your teeth for most — if not all — of your life. You can't afford to worry only about the toothache you have today, or the three cavities you got this year. And you can't rush to the dentist only when you're in pain from a cavity or an abscess. You have to look at what kind of shape your teeth are in and commit yourself to a lifetime of regular wellness care in order to keep them in your mouth as long as possible.

The same thing applies to your spine. You're going to have your spine the rest of your life. You can't just consider the backache you have today, or even the subluxations you had corrected last month. And you can't be rushing to the chiropractor when you have a medical "problem" to fix. In order to maintain good spinal health, you must commit yourself to a lifetime of wellness care.

So, the question "how many times will I have to come in to see you before I'm healthy?" is actually answered by another question that only you can answer: "How long do you wish to take good care of yourself?"

Of course, there are times when spinal nerve interference is linked to an acute health problem, such as pain or stiffness. Even though the chiropractic adjustment is not provided to treat those problems, many patients are concerned with how long their bodies will take to return to their normal functioning. Yet, even that question is hard to answer!

> **An optimist is one who sees a light where there is none. A pessimist is one who blows it out.**
>
> **— B.J. Palmer**

The CCP puts it this way:

"Individual differences in each patient and the unique circumstances of each clinical encounter preclude the formulation of 'cookbook' recommendations for frequency and duration of care." The CCP Guidelines also notes, "since the duration of care for the correction of vertebral subluxation is patient specific, frequency of visits should be based upon the reduction and eventual resolution of indicators of vertebral subluxation."

The most difficult thing about figuring out how long the corrective phase of care should last is the fact that the symptoms often disappear before the spinal nerve interference is totally corrected. A patient, for example, who comes in with terrible migraine headaches might start getting relief after only a few visits to the chiropractor. There's a temptation at that point for the patient to think he or she is healthy again, and to stop going to be adjusted.

But often, the symptoms are the last thing to appear— and the first thing to disappear — even though the body hasn't regained a fully functioning nerve system. Stop chiropractic care too soon, and the spinal nerve interference can cause subtle damage without you ever knowing it (until, unfortunately, it's too late).

Today, doctors of chiropractic use a variety of re-examination procedures to keep track of and measure their patients' progress. A general reassessment is made each visit, and a more detailed re-evaluation is usually done periodically. By comparing the results of the re-examination to the original results, the doctor can determine precisely what kind of progress the patient is making, and how well the adjustments are holding.

Re-examination is so important that the CCP made it part of their Guidelines. "The reassessment provides information necessary to perform an adjustment on a per-visit basis," the document reads. "Partial reassessment involves duplication of two or more preceding positive analytical procedures. Full reassessment involves duplication of three or more preceding positive analytical procedures... The frequency of partial and full reassessments should be at the discretion of the practitioners, consistent with the objectives of the plan of care."

Chapter 7

IN A COURT OF LAW

Experts say that the majority of medical malpractice cases could have been avoided if there had been clear communication between the patient and the doctor. Historically, doctors of chiropractic have had few legal battles with patients because they have been good communicators.

Patients say that, unlike medical doctors, chiropractors are willing to take time to explain things to their patients and don't talk down to them. They aren't in a big rush to write a prescription or send someone to the operating room. Instead, they educate their patients and, in return, listen to them.

Yet, even the best communicator can sometimes run into a brick wall. There are people so distracted by the proceedings in the chiropractic office, that they don't really listen to what the doctor or chiropractic assistant is saying. They may nod in the right places, and sign the Terms of Acceptance, but they don't really absorb what they are hearing.

One patient, who went to his chiropractor after an automobile accident, complained of headaches, soreness and fatigue. The doctor examined him and detected subluxations involving several vertebrae. After about six visits, his headaches were gone and he was feeling great. But two months later, during a regular medical checkup, he found out he had a spot on his lung — completely unrelated to the accident or the chiropractic care.

It turned out it was not cancerous, but he was furious that the chiropractor hadn't diagnosed it. "He took all those tests and X-rays. He should have seen it," he complained, completely forgetting what the doctor had explained to him about subluxations and what he would be receiving with chiropractic care.

The patient still wasn't satisfied, so he mentioned his complaint to his medical doctor, who ridiculed him for having seen a chiropractor in the first place. "If they're going to go around calling themselves doctors," he told the patient, "they ought to be able to diagnose like doctors." Encouraged by his medical doctor, the patient went to a lawyer, who urged him to sue.

By then, though, he had looked through all his paperwork from the chiropractor and found the Terms of Acceptance, which he had signed. "I guess I should have read this more carefully," he admitted to the lawyer.

However, the lawyer, who had never worked with chiropractors and did not understand the first thing about the chiropractic profession, said it didn't matter. "They can't just sign away their liability," he argued. "They are doctors and they have to be able to diagnose diseases and problems. That's what a doctor is for. They can't just say they're interested only in subluxations."

The argument didn't get very far. When the chiropractor was contacted about the possible lawsuit, he showed the patient's attorney a copy of the state licensing statute which clearly stated that the practice of a doctor of chiropractic was specifically focused on the correction of subluxation and that providing medical diagnosis and treatment was considered practicing medicine without a license.

The patient and his lawyer were subdued, but weren't ready to give up the chance for a lucrative settlement. That's when the chiropractor took out a long list of court cases and legal opinions concerning the proper scope of practice of a chiropractor, and the legitimacy of Terms of Acceptance forms.

After one look at these cases and related information, the patient and his lawyer conferred for a few minutes, then returned to apologize to the doctor and drop all of the complaints.

The state licensing statutes are usually quite clear about the limitations of chiropractic scope of practice. Kentucky says it very concisely: "Chiropractic means the science of diagnosing and adjusting the subluxations of the articulations of the human spine and its adjacent tissues."

Most other states are a bit wordier in their definitions, but the intent is generally the same. Insurance company representatives, attorneys, judges and juries often put more weight on the outcome of cases which have been decided in courts.

The cases help give a clearer picture of how the courts around the country have viewed the chiropractic profession, and how they repeatedly have upheld the obligation of chiropractors to focus solely on the diagnosis and correction of spinal nerve interference.

Let's look at a few of the more interesting or important cases.

> # We make a living by what we get; but a life by what we give.
>
> — B.J. Palmer

Daley v. Dahmer, D.C., Circuit Court for Pinellas County, Flor. (1986)

When the plaintiff, Mrs. Daley, first came to Dr. David Dahmer's practice in Florida, he gave her the same lay lecture he gave all his new patients. He explained all about chiropractic and the vertebral subluxation, and emphasized that he did not treat symptoms or conditions. His job was to detect and correct subluxations so the body could function more normally. He explained the Terms of Acceptance, and had her sign the form stating that she understood what chiropractic was about.

Two years later, after moving to Texas, she sued Dahmer for malpractice, demanding $1.5 million! Dr. Dahmer was very courageous and held fast to his principles. His insurance company tried to get him to settle the case for $40,000, and told him that if he wanted to go to trial he would have to pay any losses beyond that amount. Dr. Dahmer refused to settle the case and admit he was wrong.

During the trial, he showed the Terms of Acceptance form to the jury and gave them the same lay lecture he gave all new patients. He was found not guilty and the court ordered Mrs. Daley to "take nothing by this action."

> **You can deceive others easily; yourself, perhaps, for a time; but Innate, never.**
>
> **— B.J. Palmer**

This decision demonstrated that the Terms of Acceptance is completely legal. In addition, it confirmed that a signed form is strong evidence that the patient had no reason NOT to understand the type of care he or she was to receive and therefore will rarely — if ever — have grounds upon which to sue for medically related matters.

Cobb v. Beatty Chiropractic Clinic Lawyers weekly, No. 31860, unpublished per curiam).

In this Michigan case, a patient sued his doctor of chiropractic for failing to suspect a medical condition which later, in his opinion, needed medical treatment. The doctor neither diagnosed the problem nor referred him to a medical practitioner.

But the judge noted the Michigan Supreme Court had explained that "the legislature did not intend to authorize chiropractors to undertake differential diagnostic techniques to diagnose or rule out the existence of localized non-spinal ailments." It also interpreted the legislative actions to mean that the scope of chiropractic practice did "not include the duty to originally diagnose non-spinal ailments to determine whether they are treatable by chiropractic or whether the treatment should be done by another health-care professional."

In short, since chiropractic does not — legally or traditionally — involve the diagnosis or treatment of diseases or other medical conditions, patients cannot expect their chiropractors to discover these ailments.

People v. Beno, D.C., 422 Mich. 293. 373 N.W.2d 544 (1985).

In this case, the court determined that the "Practice of chiropractic" referred to the health care discipline which deals with "the nervous system and its relationship to the spinal column and its interrelationship with other body systems." This included diagnosis, including spinal analysis, to determine the existence of spinal subluxations or misalignments that produce spinal nerve interference, indicating the necessity for chiropractic care.

In wording it that way, it is clear the court agreed that the reason for any "diagnosis" by a chiropractor was solely to determine whether the patient had subluxations and could benefit from chiropractic care. No mention is made of any medical conditions or health problems other than subluxation.

In addition, the court held that chiropractic adjustments were given in order to establish "neural integrity utilizing the inherent recuperative powers of the body for restoration and maintenance of health."

Most significant in this case was the statement that chiropractors could use analytical instruments, nutritional advice, rehabilitative exercise and adjustment apparatus, as well as X-ray machines "for the purpose of locating spinal subluxations or misaligned vertebrae of the human spine."

Don't take yourself too damned seriously.

— B.J. Palmer

People v. Bovee. D.C.. 285 N.W. 2d 53 (Mich.Ct.App. 1979).

This case stemmed from the actions of a chiropractor who dispensed various medicines for colds, headaches, pain and nasal congestion. He also would take throat cultures and urine samples and imply to patients that he was diagnosing and treating specific health conditions.

The court said he went too far and was actually practicing medicine without a license. The reasoning was simple. State law declared that the practice of medicine means "to diagnose, treat, prevent, cure, or relieve a human disease, ailment, defect, complaint, or other condition, whether physical or mental, by attendance or advice, or by a device, diagnostic test, or other means, or to offer, undertake, attempt to do, or hold oneself out as able to do, any of these acts."

On the other hand, the Michigan law defined chiropractic as "the locating of misaligned or displaced vertebrae of the human spine, the procedure preparatory to and the adjustment by hand of such misaligned or displaced vertebrae and surrounding bones or tissues, for the restoration and maintenance of health." The statute also permitted chiropractors to use X-rays and other approved pieces of equipment during their examinations, but "solely for the purpose of locating misaligned or displaced vertebrae of the human spine and for the procedures preparatory thereto."

When Dr. Bovee began presenting himself as a medical doctor — that is, as a doctor who was involved in the diagnosis and treatment of diseases or conditions other than subluxation — he had been practicing medicine without a license.

Dowell v. Mossberg, 226 Or.173, 355 P.2d 624(1960).

Although most doctors of chiropractic do not diagnose and treat medical ailments or conditions (other than vertebral subluxations) some do attempt that kind of diagnosis and even take blood or urine samples. When they do, however, they run a big risk.

First, as was seen in a previous case, they may be found guilty of practicing medicine without a license. But even if that isn't the case, they are going to be held responsible for providing the same kind of care as medical doctors.

In other words, doctors of chiropractic who attempt full body diagnosis cannot later say they can't be held liable for a missed or inaccurate diagnosis because they are chiropractors. If they are going to try to act like medical doctors, they are going to be held to the same standard as medical doctors.

That's the conclusion of this case, in which a doctor took several urine samples of his patient, and made notations in his records of the sugar content. In one, he noted a high sugar concentration, which is one of the things to look for when testing for diabetes.

This doctor was obviously not looking for spinal nerve interference. He would have had no reason to remark the sugar content of the patient's urine unless he was looking for specific ailments. And, there is no evidence he ever told the patient that he wasn't trying to diagnose disease. In addition, he did not use any kind of informed consent or Terms of Acceptance form.

It was only logical that the patient would think this doctor was giving her a thorough medical exam, complete with urine tests. When she later found she had diabetes, she was irate. Why didn't the doctor — seeing the first suspicious signs of possible diabetes — do additional tests? At the very least, why didn't he tell her about the test results and refer her to a medical doctor? If he was going to present himself as a "medical" doctor, he should be responsible for proper diagnosis.

The court agreed, noting that chiropractors who clearly

explain that they focus solely on the detection and correction of the vertebral subluxation, "should not be held, in a malpractice case, to a degree of science or skill which (they have) never claimed."

However, "if a practitioner holds himself out as a diagnostician and undertakes to examine all sufferers who present themselves, he is in competition with those who are licensed and recognized as competent to diagnose and treat a wide variety of human ailments. When the practitioner so undertakes, he must exercise the same degree of care and skill as those with whom he seeks to compete."

In this case, the defendant actually claimed he was capable of diagnosing diabetes as well as other ailments, saying that when he detected illnesses, he normally referred the patient to a medical doctor. The court noted that, if chiropractors claim to be able to diagnose diabetes or other ailments, their patients have the right to expect them to have the same degree of skill and care as medical doctors in the diagnostic procedure.

In addition, the court said it would be perfectly acceptable to have medical doctors testify against such chiropractors in court, something that usually isn't allowed when the case involves a subluxation-based chiropractor.

> # Any method which treats effects is the practice of medicine.
>
> ## — B.J. Palmer

Spunt v. Fowinkle, 572 S.W.2d 259, Tenn.Ct.App. (1 978).

Here's another case of a chiropractor who forgot the true purpose of chiropractic. Instead of focusing on the detection of the spinal nerve interference, he decided he was going to offer medical procedures such as drawing blood and taking Pap smears.

Yet, the Tennessee statute under which he was licensed clearly stated, "Chiropractic is defined as the science of palpating, analyzing and adjusting the articulations of the human spinal column and adjacent tissues by hand." State law also said that "Any person shall be regarded as practicing medicine within the meaning of this chapter who shall treat, or profess to treat, operate on, or prescribe for any physical ailment or physical injury to or deformity of another."

There is no need to draw blood or do a Pap smear in order to analyze the spine and detect spinal nerve interference. There's only one reason that this doctor would have carried out those procedures (and he admitted as much during his testimony): to diagnose diseases such as cancer and make treatment recommendations based on his findings.

> ## And some chiropractors want to give a pill as a substitute for Innate.
>
> ### — B.J. Palmer

What he was doing, then, was playing medical doctor, and the court found that he went beyond the practice of chiropractic and invaded the field of medicine.

One particularly interesting aspect of this case was the fact that the court said there was, technically, nothing in the law which prohibited the doctor from doing a Pap smear or drawing blood. If either or both of these procedures were clearly for the purpose of detecting spinal nerve interference or determining a chiropractic program of care for subluxation correction, he would have been in the clear. But the doctor's purpose clearly was to diagnose disease, which meant he was crossing the line separating chiropractic from medicine.

Kerkman v. Hintz, 142 Wis.2d 404, 4178 N.W.2d 795 (1988).

This case again points out the very clear differences between chiropractic and medical practice.

Wisconsin state code stated that the practice of chiropractic included "examination, counsel and advice with respect to the diagnosis and/or analysis of any interference with normal nerve transmission, expression and the correction thereof by a chiropractic adjustment to remove the interference as a cause of disease, without the use of drugs or surgery." In other words, the detection and correction of vertebral subluxations.

The code also added: "The science of chiropractic is based on the premise that disease or abnormal function can be caused by abnormal nerve impulse transmission... due to compression, traction, pressure or irritation upon nerves, as the result of bony segments, especially of the spine or contiguous structures, either deviating from juxtaposition and/or functioning in an abnormal manner so as to irritate nerves or their receptors."

An expert witness testified that chiropractors do not treat or diagnose disease, but focus solely on the analysis and correction of subluxation whereas medical doctors are concerned with the diagnosis and treatment of the diseased area through the use of drugs and surgery or other techniques. Clearly, two very different and distinct professions.

That's why the court found that chiropractors who abide by the definition of chiropractic and maintain a subluxation-based practice, cannot be held responsible for making medical diagnoses or giving medical treatments.

DEFINING CHIROPRACTIC

We could go on listing more cases which arrived at similar conclusions, but even these few show clearly that chiropractic is not medicine and medicine is not chiropractic. The two are totally different professions, with different philosophies, purposes and procedures.

Chiropractors have to make sure patients understand the difference and have the proper expectations about the care they will

> ## Men of principle are the principal men.
> ### — B.J. Palmer

receive. If patients aren't clear about what to expect from chiropractic (or, worse, if the doctor of chiropractic doesn't seem clear about this!) there can be serious consequences.

But all this could easily be avoided by the use of effective patient education tools and proper forms such as the Terms of Acceptance, and Report of Unusual Findings.

As a patient, you have to shoulder part of the responsibility as well. You have to make sure you understand the differences and don't go to a chiropractor expecting him or her to diagnose your ailments and treat you! Instead, you need to find a chiropractor who shares your understanding that chiropractic is for the detection and correction of vertebral subluxation and the spinal nerve interference it entails — and that living subluxation-free is the best thing you can possibly do for your health!

> **Conditions change, and our attitude towards them has changed, but principles remain the same.**
>
> **— B.J. Palmer**

Chapter 8

WHO REALLY
KNOWS ABOUT
CHIROPRACTIC?

I n May 1998, the *Journal of the American Medical Association* reported that two out of every five Americans surveyed have used chiropractic or another form of non-medical health care either along with, or in place of drug or surgical treatment from the allopathic medical profession. This is, of course, rather alarming for all those connected with medicine — doctors, hospitals, drug companies, medical equipment manufacturers and researchers, all of whom make tons of money from illness.

This news about the defection of 40% of the population away from medicine came just months after The National Patient Safety Foundation released the results of several studies conducted by Lucian Leape, M.D. of the Harvard School of Public Health.

Published in October 1997, the reports estimated that well over 3 million people have been killed or injured by medical errors. The Feb. 28, 1998 issue of *The Lancet*, a British medical journal, reported that during the past 10 years, the number of people who have died from medical drug errors has nearly tripled.

Deaths linked to chiropractic or other non-medical health care fields are so rare they are considered oddities which can't even be represented by meaningful statistics.

Yet, medical doctors routinely "warn" patients not to go to any non-medical professional, except on their referral (which doesn't happen very often!) In fact, most medical personnel are so against other forms of health care that many patients hide the fact that they are seeing a chiropractor or other practitioner for fear of getting a scolding from the offended M.D.

Incredibly, many people in our society still maintain a blind trust in the medical profession, despite the increasing number of reports showing it to be riddled with greed, incompetence and prejudice against other professions. If their medical doctor says chiropractic is dangerous, or ineffective, or worthless, they listen without question.

The truth is, it's the opinion of a medical doctor on the art and science of chiropractic that's worthless. Think of it this way. If you had electrical work done in your house, would you ask your plumber to make sure the electrician did everything right? Would you go to your bank teller to find out if your car mechanic fixed your brakes properly? Or, for that matter, would you ask your chiropractor to make sure your optometrist's prescription was correct?

Of course not. Each profession has its own specialty. Experts in one field cannot be expected to pass judgment on or give advice about the work of another professional. They might give their personal opinions, based on their own experience or their biases one way or the other, but that free advice is worth what you pay for it — nothing!

So it is with medical doctors. They have their own profession, with their specific education, training, and experience. What they learn in school and do in practice has nothing to do with chiropractic. They therefore are not competent to give their professional opinions about the effectiveness or safety of chiropractic care.

Here, too, the courts agree.

Years ago, before the legal system stepped in and recognized that the AMA and the other medical organizations were conducting an illegal campaign to destroy chiropractic, it was commonplace to have physicians testify against chiropractors in court. But, they always spoke from their own perspective as medical doctors and attempted to apply medical definitions and standards to the doctor of chiropractic and the chiropractic profession, as though the two professions were identical.

Finally, however, the courts decided that any professional has the right to be judged by his or her peers, that is, members of the same profession. Today, when someone tries to pit a medical doctor against a chiropractor in court, the D.C. has plenty of legal case precedents to rely on to insure that doesn't happen.

The following are a few of the many legal cases which prove that medical doctors are not qualified to give professional opinions about chiropractic care.

> # Sincerity alone, therefore, is not enough; it must be wise or it may be diabolical.
>
> ## — B.J. Palmer

Sheppard v. Firth. D.C., 215 Or. 268, 334 P.2d 190(1959).

In this case, a medical doctor was allowed to testify that the care given to the plaintiff by the doctor of chiropractic she was suing was not proper and had resulted in aggravating the plaintiff's condition.

On appeal, however, the appellate court said this wasn't right. The principle that doctors have the right to be judged ONLY by the standards of the field to which they belong applies to drugless practitioners as well as physicians. It was unfair to let a medical doctor make value judgments regarding the care provided by a doctor of chiropractic.

The higher court also decided that the medical doctor shouldn't have been allowed to testify as to the value of a neurocalometer (an instrument used by chiropractors to detect subluxation) since medical doctors have no training or experience with the device.

Sutton v. Cook, 254 Or. 116, 458 P.2d 402 (1969).

The judges in this case were very clear about their position when they stated, "We have held that a drugless healer is entitled to have his conduct in the treatment of his patients tested by standards applicable to the school or system to which he belongs and not by the standards of medical practice."

> **Be sure you're right — then force the fight.**
>
> **— B.J. Palmer**

Boudreaux v. Panger, D.C.. 481 So.2d 1382 (La.Ct.App. 1986).

In this case, the chiropractor had to face two orthopedic surgeons, who testified that he had not provided adequate medical care. The court noted that "While the orthopedic surgeons certainly are experts in their own field, neither physician admitted to any expertise or skill in manipulation of the vertebrae as defined for chiropractors... We cannot agree that the medical testimony was sufficient to show either a standard of chiropractic care or a negligent standard of chiropractic care." The chiropractor won the case.

Morgan v. Hill. 663 S.W.2d 232. Ky.Ct.App. (1984).

In this case, the court said that a medical doctor was as qualified as a chiropractor to testify as to the cause of any injury. But, the decision added, a medical doctor "may not testify to the chiropractor's standard of care, however, because he does not have the appropriate training and experience to determine what constitutes chiropractic malpractice."

Stackhouse v. Scanlon. M.D. 576 N.E.2d 635 (Ind.Ct.App. 1991).

This case deals with the other side of the coin. Just as M.D.s are not qualified to testify about chiropractic cases, D.C.s are not qualified to render professional opinions about medical treatment. The reasoning remains the same: the two professions are totally different!

Taormina v. Goodman, 406 N.Y.S. 2d 350 (N.Y.App.Div. 1978).

This case also emphasizes that, as the court put it, "the practice of chiropractic is separate and distinct from the practice of medicine… so that a physician's standard of care can no longer be considered controlling upon a chiropractor in the practice of his profession." However, the judge added an important caveat: "Of course, a physician's standard would apply where a chiropractor departs from the restrictions placed upon the practice of his profession… and ventures into the practice of medicine."

What the public thinks

The courts understand fully that physicians are not qualified to render opinions about chiropractic care, but the public is often fooled into thinking that medical doctors know it all!

They will, for instance, go to their medical doctor for nutritional advice, even though a report released by the College of Physicians and Surgeons at Columbia-Presbyterian Medical Center Office of Public Health in April 1997 noted that only 29 out of 129 U.S. medical schools required any courses in nutrition— and 21 didn't offer any!

In the report, Richard Deckelbaum, M.D., director of the Institute of Human Nutrition at Columbia University said, "Education of physicians on nutrition-related matters is abysmal… clinical nutrition has been overlooked because it cannot be identified with any particular physiological system in the body, as most medical specialities can. "Obviously, one of the last people to go to for nutritional advice is your medical doctor!

What's even more startling is that some people go to their medical doctor for advice on chiropractic or other forms of alternative health care. Not only are M.D.s lacking in any training or experience in these disciplines, most have been indoctrinated into thinking that anything non-medical is either a fraud or a threat.

When you want advice or information about chiropractic, do what the courts do — forget the M.D.s and go to the only practitioners who understand the profession: doctors of chiropractic!

Chapter 9

CHIROPRACTIC FAQS
(FREQUENTLY ASKED QUESTIONS)

The computer and Internet revolution have given us a great many wonderful innovations. One of the best is the presence of files called FAQs — "Frequently Asked Questions." These files help answer a lot of the questions people have about any topic. So, we thought it was fitting to include a chiropractic FAQ in this book.

Q. I now understand about vertebral subluxations. But how do I know if I have any which require chiropractic care?

A. The only sure way to know if you are subluxated is to schedule an examination with a doctor of chiropractic. However, there are several simple tests which you can give yourself or members of your family. Although these aren't as accurate as the ones your doctor will use, they may give you early indications of possible subluxations. For your convenience, we've included some of these tests in the appendix of this book, along with a test "score" card. If any of the tests reveal the possibility of subluxations, take the card to your chiropractor on your first visit.

Q. If subluxations can cause all kinds of physical problems, how can I be subluxated but not be sick or have any symptoms?

A. Your definition of healthy might be incomplete. Just because you don't feel sick or have symptoms, doesn't necessarily mean you're healthy. How many times have you heard of a person who died suddenly of a heart attack? His friends are shocked.

"But he was so healthy," they say. Was he? If he was healthy, with a strong and healthy heart and a good nerve supply, would he have had a heart attack and died? Usually, in such cases, the person is not healthy — just healthy looking.

Most bodily functions go on all the time without you ever being aware of them. You normally aren't conscious of when your organs are working correctly and you may not know it when they aren't — until it's too late.

Remember when you first learned, back in grade school, that the earth was spinning around at an incredible speed. If you're like most kids, you went out into the school yard and stood still and tried to feel the earth spinning. How could it possibly be happening if you didn't feel it? Of course, the scientific evidence was so overwhelming that there could be no room for doubt that this unbelievable phenomenon was true.

> Coming together is a beginning.
> Keeping together is progress.
> Working together is success.
> — B.J. Palmer

None of us today, as adults, doubt for a second that the earth is spinning — even if we can't feel it underfoot. Yet, we have trouble believing interference in our nerve system can cause health problems in the rest of our body, or that we can be very UNhealthy and not show any symptoms — despite the overwhelming evidence.

Q. Am I signing away any of my rights as a patient if I sign a Terms of Acceptance form?

A. Absolutely not! The doctor of chiropractic is responsible for giving you safe, proper chiropractic care.

However, by signing the Terms of Acceptance, you are acknowledging that you will hold your doctor responsible for chiropractic — NOT medical — care and that you understand the difference. It is a way for you and your doctor to make sure the care you receive matches the expectations you have.

Q. On my Report of Unusual Findings, my doctor noted something unusual but she didn't tell me what disease it could be or if I should see a medical doctor or a specialist. Why not?

A. In order for your doctor of chiropractic to give you details about what medical condition you may have, or even figure out what kind of health care professional to send you to, she would have to make a medical diagnosis of the problem. As a chiropractor, she is not trained to do that kind of diagnosis, and the scope of practice laws in her state may not even permit her to do it. You wouldn't want her to make a "guess" about something that important, would you?

Q. I went to a chiropractor for headaches last year but left because they stopped after just two sessions, even though my doctor urged me to continue care. Now the headaches are back but, after learning about chiropractic, I'm a little embarrassed to go back to him. I live in a small town and we have only one D.C. Should I ignore my embarrassment, or go to a medical doctor instead?

A. Swallow your pride and go back to your chiropractor. Believe me, he'll understand and be glad you've decided to seek help. But keep in mind that he's NOT treating your headaches. They are merely symptoms of something wrong in your system. Your chiropractor will see if you have spinal nerve interference and adjust you if you do. Your body's inner wisdom will work on the headaches.

Q. My chiropractor is what you'd call subluxation-based, but he also gives me nutritional advice and even told me where to buy a better pillow! What has this got to do with subluxations?

A. Many things can cause subluxations, including poor nutrition, improper posture, physical or emotional stress, and even bad

To restore normal transmission of mental impulse to peripheral function is to practice chiropractic.

— B.J. Palmer

sleeping positions! Your doctor is trying to get you to do whatever you can so your adjustments will hold and you will prevent future spinal nerve interference. The only time patients have to worry is when their chiropractor gives them advice about how to relieve specific symptoms or treat diseases.

Q. I am a chiropractic assistant in a busy metropolitan clinic. All of our doctors are strictly subluxation-based and we place a strong emphasis on education. Unfortunately, one of the doctors here was sued recently by a patient who claimed the D.C. hadn't diagnosed a head injury he'd suffered in a car accident months before. The doctor met with a lawyer recommended by his malpractice insurance company, but he doesn't seem to know anything about chiropractic. He seems to think it's just another medical therapy. I hate to butt into the doctor's business, but what should he do?

A. Whenever a legal matter comes up, subluxation-based chiropractors need to find an attorney who understands exactly what chiropractic is all about. The lawyer has to know about various court decisions that will help prove the D.C.'s case. This may take some "shopping around," or even education. (For starters, make sure the lawyer has a copy of this book!) An attorney who doesn't understand subluxation-based chiropractic cannot be expected to defend a subluxation-based chiropractor.

Also, the doctor should probably re-examine his malpractice insurance company. Unfortunately, some policies are written by companies which do not support subluxation-based chiropractic and will not do anything to help their policy holders fight unfounded lawsuits. Only a company like Chiropractic Benefit Services, which was specifically started to serve the subluxation-based chiropractic community, has the knowledge to work for the rights of these doctors.

By the way, your doctor is very lucky to have a C.A. as caring and committed as you are. Never worry about "butting in" when it comes to showing how interested you are in your doctor's practice. I'm sure he appreciates it.

Q. Recently, I went to a doctor of chiropractic who told me I had chronic sinusitis and needed 14 weekly treatments to cure it. I'm tempted, since the medical doctors haven't been able to do anything about the condition, but I'm worried, too. It seems as though this goes against everything you're saying.

A. Chiropractic is a very diverse profession. As we mentioned in Chapter 3, some doctors of chiropractic have recently begun trespassing into medical territory. They tell patients that they can diagnose and treat specific diseases, and use many of the tests and "props" of their medical counterparts. We are not going to condemn these doctors, but they are considered by most of their colleagues as being outside the mainstream of the profession. Since they hold themselves out as medical practitioners, they also run the risk of being judged by medical standards.

In addition, their patients' expectations will be different than

---

> Success depends upon desire backed by will, expressed in intelligent and persistent action.
>
> — B.J. Palmer

the expectations of a person seeing a subluxation-based doctor. If any patients later discover the chiropractic physician did not properly or thoroughly diagnose their current and potential health problems, they will be treated in a court of law as though they were practicing medicine. Of course, they may also face charges of practicing medicine without a license, but that's another matter.

If you go to a doctor of chiropractic who diagnoses a specific disease, and "prescribes" a particular program of treatment to treat or cure it, then you have the right to expect that doctor to give you the same level of medical care as a medical doctor. Of course, if you really want medical care, you'd probably have continued going to medical doctors in the first place. But you know from personal experience that didn't work very well.

Instead, it sounds as though you're looking for a non-medical alternative to the routine medical response of drugs and surgery. We'd recommend finding a subluxation-based doctor who can get to the root of your problem by checking for spinal nerve interference. You might find that once your body is able to enjoy a more normal nerve supply, it may take care of the sinus-related symptoms you're experiencing. If it does, thank your new chiropractor — and your own body!

Q. I've heard a lot of horror stories about the medical profession in general and hospitals in particular. But it's hard to get the facts. Any suggestions?

A. In recent years, medicine has become big business. Pharmaceutical companies and huge health care conglomerates have taken over and make most of their "health care" decisions based on what is the most profitable. Because they account for a sizeable portion of the advertising revenue on television, radio and in our publications, they can make sure most of the negative information never reaches the public.

But there are several excellent books which provide evidence of the problems we face in this country because of the medical monopoly. You might start with Dr. Terry Rondberg's book, "Under the Influence of Modern Medicine," which fully documents some of the abuses in this system.

> **Living should be a continuous letting go of education of the past to discover great depths in Innate's future.**
>
> **— B.J. Palmer**

Definitions

ADJUSTMENT: The specific application of forces used to facilitate the body's correction of spinal nerve interference.

CHIROPRACTIC: A primary health care profession in which professional responsibility and authority are focused on the anatomy of the spine and immediate articulation, and the condition of spinal nerve interference. It is also a practice that encompasses educating, advising about, and addressing spinal nerve interference.

CHIROPRACTIC DIAGNOSIS: A comprehensive process of evaluation of the spinal column and its immediate articulations to determine the presence of spinal nerve interference and other conditions that may contraindicate chiropractic procedures.

CHIROPRACTIC PRACTICE OBJECTIVE: The professional practice objective of chiropractic is to correct spinal nerve interference in a safe, effective manner. The correction is not considered to be a specific cure for any particular symptom or disease. It is applicable to any patient who exhibits spinal nerve interference regardless of the presence or absence of symptoms or disease.

DIS-EASE: The word *disease* is a combination of *dis* and *ease*. *Dis* is a prefix meaning "apart from." It follows then that dis-ease is nothing more than a lack of comfort, a loss of harmony in the system. Chiropractors believe that instead of treating disease with chemicals and invasive procedures, whenever possible, they should address dis-ease with the reduction or elimination of spinal nerve interference, thereby giving the patient a chance to recover naturally before resorting to drugs and surgery.

HEALTH: A state of optimal physical, mental and social

well being, not merely the absence of disease or infirmity.

MANIPULATION: The forceful passive movement of a joint beyond its active limit of motion. It doesn't imply the use of precision, specificity or the correction of spinal nerve interference. Therefore, it is not synonymous with chiropractic adjustment.

MEDICAL DIAGNOSIS: Procedures that provide information about disease processes for the selection of treatment.

THE MAJOR PREMISE IN CHIROPRACTIC: A universal intelligence is in all matter and continually gives to it all its properties and actions, thus maintaining it in existence.

VITALISM: The doctrine that teaches that in living organisms, life is caused and sustained by a vital principle distinct from all physical and chemical forces. It also teaches that life is, at least in part, self-determining and self-evolving.

VERTEBRAL SUBLUXATION: A misalignment of one or more of the vertebrae in the spinal column, which causes alteration of nerve functions and interference to the transmission of mental impulses resulting in a lessening of the body's innate ability to express its maximum health potential. Also referred to as spinal nerve interference.

APPENDIX

12 WAYS TO TEST FOR SPINAL NERVE INTERFERENCE

To enjoy optimum physical and emotional well being, our bodies have to be working properly, with a nerve supply that can relay electrical impulses from the brain to every organ and cell — and back again — without interference or distortion.

If anything interferes with this nerve supply, we can experience a variety of responses including pain, stiffness, a specific illness, reduced immune response, or dysfunction in one or more of the body's other life support systems.

If we're lucky, the interference will trigger symptoms which act as "warning signals," telling us something is wrong. Yet, too often, the effects are so subtle we don't realize anything's wrong until it's too late. Many serious health problems can be traced to the devastating effects of spinal nerve interference which weakens organs without displaying outward signs.

Spinal nerve interference — also called vertebral subluxation — is a misalignment of bones along the spinal column. Nerves branching off the spinal cord from the brain pass through small openings between the interlocking bones and travel throughout the body. When the bones are out of their normal positions — which can happen due to injury, bad posture, muscle imbalance, or

93

even emotional or chemical stress — the subluxation will cause interference in the flow of nerve energy.

The only safe and effective way to correct a subluxation is to go to a chiropractor for an adjustment. This is the term for the specific application of forces used to facilitate the body's correction of spinal nerve interference. Doctors of chiropractic are the only health professionals who have the extensive training and experience necessary to detect and correct vertebral subluxations.

However, here are 12 easy spinal exam procedures which may indicate the presence of vertebral subluxations. It is best to perform each of these tests on yourself each month. To safeguard the health of family members — including children — they should be tested as well. If you obtain a positive result on any of the tests, you should see your family chiropractor as soon as possible.

Range of Motion

For each of the following tests, stand in an upright, relaxed position. Your movements should be slow and gentle — never use jerky or forceful motions. If you cannot turn or bend the full distance, mark the appropriate box in the chart. If you experience any pain or discomfort, check that box as well.

Test 1: Rotation — Turn your head slowly to the right, then to the left. Do not move your upper body. You should be able to turn so that your chin is nearly parallel with your shoulder.

Test 2: Lateral Flexion — Bend your head slowly to the right, then to the left. Do not raise your shoulders. You should be able to bring your ears within an inch or two of your shoulders.

Test 3: Flexion/Extension — Bend your head slowly to the front, then to the back. You should be able to look straight up and straight down.

Test 4: Rotation — Turn, from the waist, to your left, then to your right. Do not move your feet or hips and keep your head in line with your upper body. You should be able to turn about 45 degrees in each direction.

Test 5: Lateral Flexion — Bend from the waist to the right, then to the left. You should be able to bend about 45 degrees in each direction.

Test 6: Flexion/Extension — Bend forward, then backwards, from the waist. Keep your back straight, your head in line with your upper body, and do not bend your knees. You should be able to bend forward until you are parallel with the floor, and backward far enough to be able to look straight up.

Postural Checks

For these tests, you'll need to stand in front of a full length mirror or have a partner examine you. Close your eyes, take a few breaths and "shake" all the tension from your body. When you feel totally relaxed, open your eyes and remain perfectly still. Examine your reflection but don't attempt to "correct" any postural problems — just note them. You might find it easier to first make several straight lines — horizontal lines and one full length vertical line on the mirror surface with tape, soap, or other easy-to-clean substances. Compare the "line" of your body to these lines and determine if you are parallel to the mirror lines, or if you are out of balance. Mark the appropriate box for each test in the chart.

Test 7: Midline — draw an imaginary line vertically through your body, from the top of your head, through your nose, chin, belly button and down to your feet. Is this line parallel to the vertical line on the mirror or is it out of balance?

Test 8: Ears — draw an imaginary line horizontally through your ears. Is it parallel to the lines on the mirror or is it out of balance?

95

Test 9: Shoulders — draw an imaginary line across your shoulders. Is it parallel to the lines on the mirror or is it out of balance?

Test 10: Waistline — draw an imaginary line through your waistline. Is it parallel to the lines on the mirror or is it out of balance?

Leg Length Check

Test 11: For this test, you will need a test partner. Lie on your back on the floor (or other firm, flat surface). Make sure your body is as straight and relaxed as possible. Test partner instructions: "cup" the subject's heels in your hands, with your fingers on the outside and your thumbs on the bottom of the heel, pointing toward each other. Press the feet together and push them up slightly (toward the subject's head) with equal thumb pressure on each foot. Now, look down over the feet and see if one leg appears slightly shorter than the other. Look carefully, since the difference may only be a fraction of an inch. If there is a difference, note which leg looks shorter and mark it on the chart.

Palpation

Test 12: This test also requires a test partner. Lie face down in a relaxed position. Test partner instructions: With the blunt ends of your fingers (not the tips, but the fleshy part where the fingerprints are), press on the "bumps" along the subject's spine. Use moderate pressure — about the same amount you'd use to check the ripeness of a melon. Work from the base of the skull to the lower back, feeling for each individual spinal bone. If the subject experiences any tenderness, soreness or discomfort, circle the spot on the spinal chart which comes closest to the place you touched.

Test Results

	Normal	Restricted	Pain
Test 1:	☐	☐	☐
Test 2:	☐	☐	☐
Test 3:	☐	☐	☐
Test 4:	☐	☐	☐
Test 5:	☐	☐	☐
Test 6:	☐	☐	☐

	Balanced	Imbalanced
Test 7:	☐	☐
Test 8:	☐	☐
Test 9:	☐	☐
Test 10:	☐	☐

	Equal Length	Short Rt. Leg	Short Lt. Leg
Test 11:	☐	☐	☐

Test 12: Cirlce level of Column A below if it is tender or painful when palpated:

If any of these tests indicate restricted motion, pain or tenderness, imbalance, or a short leg, see a doctor of chiropractic immediately.

YOUR NERVE SYSTEM

A: The names of the vertebrae and nerves in the spine.   B: The areas known to receive nerve fibers from these nerves.

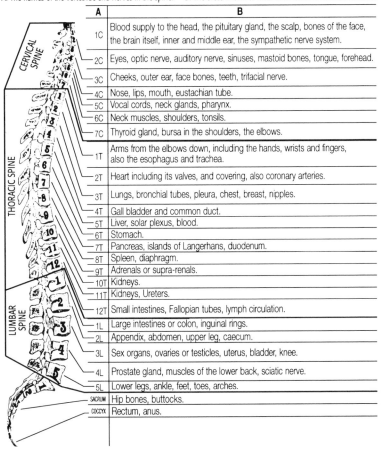

A	B
1C	Blood supply to the head, the pituitary gland, the scalp, bones of the face, the brain itself, inner and middle ear, the sympathetic nerve system.
2C	Eyes, optic nerve, auditory nerve, sinuses, mastoid bones, tongue, forehead.
3C	Cheeks, outer ear, face bones, teeth, trifacial nerve.
4C	Nose, lips, mouth, eustachian tube.
5C	Vocal cords, neck glands, pharynx.
6C	Neck muscles, shoulders, tonsils.
7C	Thyroid gland, bursa in the shoulders, the elbows.
1T	Arms from the elbows down, including the hands, wrists and fingers, also the esophagus and trachea.
2T	Heart including its valves, and covering, also coronary arteries.
3T	Lungs, bronchial tubes, pleura, chest, breast, nipples.
4T	Gall bladder and common duct.
5T	Liver, solar plexus, blood.
6T	Stomach.
7T	Pancreas, islands of Langerhans, duodenum.
8T	Spleen, diaphragm.
9T	Adrenals or supra-renals.
10T	Kidneys.
11T	Kidneys, Ureters.
12T	Small intestines, Fallopian tubes, lymph circulation.
1L	Large intestines or colon, inguinal rings.
2L	Appendix, abdomen, upper leg, caecum.
3L	Sex organs, ovaries or testicles, uterus, bladder, knee.
4L	Prostate gland, muscles of the lower back, sciatic nerve.
5L	Lower legs, ankle, feet, toes, arches.
SACRUM	Hip bones, buttocks.
COCCYX	Rectum, anus.

97

A message to Doctors of Chiropractic:

Chiropractic Benefit Services Malpractice Program supports chiropractors practicing non-allopathic, subluxation-based chiropractic. CBS is the largest financial contributor supporting the development of the Council on Chiropractic Practice guidelines. These guidelines are the only subluxation- and evidence-based guidelines in the world.

CBS is also funding research that we anticipate will prove correcting vertebral subluxations improves immune function. With CBS, you not only protect yourself, you support chiropractic as a whole. Call 1-800-883-0412 to find out more.

> **The love you give away is the love you keep.**
>
> **— B.J. Palmer**

Introduction and Methodology

The Council on Chiropractic Practice

In the summer of 1995, chiropractic history was made in Phoenix, Arizona with the formation of the Council on Chiropractic Practice (CCP). The meeting was attended by an interdisciplinary assembly of distinguished chiropractors, medical physicians, basic scientists, attorneys, and consumer representatives.

The CCP is an apolitical, non-profit organization. It is not affiliated with any other chiropractic association. The CCP represents a grassroots movement to produce practice guidelines which serve the needs of the consumer, and are consistent with "real world" chiropractic practice.

The mission of the CCP is "To develop evidence-based guidelines, conduct research and perform other functions that will enhance the practice of chiropractic for the benefit of the consumer."

Evidence-Based Practice

Evidence-based clinical practice is defined as "The conscientious, explicit, and judicious use of the current best evidence in making decisions about the care of individual patients... (it) is not restricted to randomized trials and meta-analyses. It involves tracking down the best external evidence with which to answer our clinical questions." [1]

This concept was embraced by the Association of Chiropractic Colleges in its first position paper. This paper stated:

> Chiropractic is concerned with the preservation and restoration of health, and focuses particular attention on the subluxation. A subluxation is a complex of functional and/or structural and/or pathological articular changes that compromise neural integrity and may influence organ system function and general health.
> A subluxation is evaluated, diagnosed, and managed through the use of chiropractic procedures based on the best available rational and empirical evidence. [2]

The CCP has developed practice guidelines for vertebral subluxation with the active participation of field doctors, consultants, seminar leaders, and technique experts. In addition, the Council has utilized the services of interdisciplinary experts in the Agency for Health Care Policy and Research (AHCPR) guidelines development, research design, literature review, law, clinical assessment, and clinical chiropractic.

100

Guideline Development Process

In harmony with these general principles, the CCP has created a multidisciplinary panel, supported by staff, and led by a project director. The guidelines were produced with input from methodologists familiar with guidelines development.

The first endeavor of the panel was to analyze available scientific evidence revolving around a model which depicts the safest and most efficacious delivery of chiropractic care to the consumer. A contingent of panelists, chosen for their respective skills, directed the critical review of numerous studies and other evidence.

Since the guideline process is one of continuing evolution, new evidence will be considered at periodic meetings to update the model of care defined by the guideline.

The panel gathered in a second meeting to interview technique developers to ascertain the degree to which their procedures can be expressed in an evidence-based format. Individuals representing over thirty-five named techniques participated. Others made written submissions to the panel. The technique developers presented the best available evidence they had to substantiate their protocols and assessment methods.

A primary goal of the panel is to stimulate and encourage field practitioners to adapt their practices to improve patient outcomes. To achieve this objective, it was necessary to involve as many practitioners as possible in the development of workable guidelines.

Consistent with the recommendations of AHCPR, an "open forum" was held where any interested individual could participate. Practitioners offered their opinions and insights in regard to the progress of the panel. Field practitioners who were unable to attend the "open forum" session were encouraged to make written submissions. Consumer and attorney participants offered their input. A meeting was held with chiropractic consultants to secure their participation.

After sorting and evaluating the evidence gathered in the literature review, technique forum, written comments, and open forum, the initial draft of the guideline was prepared. It was distributed to the panel for review and criticism. A revised draft was prepared based upon this input.

International input from the field was obtained when the working draft guideline document was submitted to 195 peer reviewers in 12 countries.

After incorporation of the suggestions of the reviewers, a final draft was presented to the panel for approval. This document was then submitted for proofreading and typesetting.

The purpose of these guidelines is to provide the doctor of chiropractic with a "user friendly" compendium of recommendations based upon the best available evidence. It is designed to facilitate, not replace, clinical judgment.

As Sackett wrote, "External clinical evidence can inform, but can never replace, individual clinical expertise, and it is this expertise that decides whether the external evidence applies to the individual patient at all and, if so, how it should be integrated into a clinical decision. Similarly, any external guideline must be integrated with individual clinical expertise in deciding whether and how it matches the patient's clinical state, predicament, and preferences, and thereby whether it should be applied." [1]

The most compelling reason for creating, disseminating, and utilizing clinical practice guidelines is to improve the quality of health care.

1. Sackett DL. Editorial: Evidence-based medicine. Spine 1998; 23(10):1085.

2. Position paper #1. Association of Chiropractic Colleges. July 1996.

Ratings and Categories of Evidence

Ratings

Established. Accepted as appropriate for use in chiropractic practice for the indications and applications stated.

Investigational. Further study is warranted. Evidence is equivocal, or insufficient to justify a rating of "established."

Inappropriate. Insufficient favorable evidence exists to support the use of this procedure in chiropractic practice.

Categories of Evidence

E: Expert opinion based on clinical experience, basic science rationale, and/or individual case studies. Where appropriate, this category includes legal opinions.

L: Literature support in the form of reliability and validity studies, observational studies, "pre-post" studies, and/or multiple case studies. Where appropriate, this category includes case law.

C: Controlled studies, including randomized and non-randomized clinical trials of acceptable quality.

Disclaimer

These guidelines are for informational purposes. Utilization of these guidelines is voluntary. They are not intended to replace the clinical judgement of the chiropractor. It is acknowledged that alternative practices are possible and may be preferable under certain clinical conditions. The appropriateness of a given procedure must be determined by the judgement of the practitioner and the needs and preferences of the individual patient.

It is not the purpose or intent of these guidelines to provide legal advice, or to supplant any statutes, rules, and regulations of a government body having jurisdiction over the practice of chiropractic.

These guidelines address vertebral subluxation in chiropractic practice, and do not purport to include all procedures which are permitted by law in the practice of chiropractic. Lack of inclusion of a procedure in these guidelines does not necessarily mean that the procedure is inappropriate for use in the practice of chiropractic.

Participation in the guideline development process does not necessarily imply agreement with the final product. This includes persons who participated in the technique conference, leadership conference, open forum, and peer review process. Listing of names acknowledge participation only, not necessarily approval or endorsement.

The guidelines reflect the consensus of the panel, which gave final approval to the recommendations.

1 History and Chiropractic Examination

CASE HISTORY

RECOMMENDATION

A thorough case history should precede the initiation of chiropractic care. The elements of this history should include general information, reason for seeking chiropractic care, onset and duration of any symptomatic problem, family history, past health history, occupational history, and social history.

Rating: Established

Evidence: E, L

Commentary

The purpose of the case history is to elicit information which might reveal salient points concerning the patient's spinal and general health that may lead the chiropractor to elect appropriate examination procedures. The case history may provide information which will assist the chiropractor in determining the safety and appropriateness of chiropractic care as well as the nature of additional analytical procedures to be performed. History taking is considered a key element of quality patient care necessary for effective doctor-patient communication and improved patient health outcomes.[1-4] Verbal, nonverbal and cognitive assessment are also included in the patient history. The chiropractic case history should emphasize eliciting information relevant to the etiology and clinical manifestations of vertebral subluxation.

CHIROPRACTIC EXAMINATION

RECOMMENDATION

The initial chiropractic examination shall include a case history and an assessment for the presence of vertebral subluxation, which, if present, is to be noted with regard to location and character. A review of systems may be conducted at the discretion of the practitioner, consistent with individual training and applicable state laws.

105

Reassessments may be conducted periodically throughout a course of chiropractic care to assess patient progress. Such reassessments typically emphasize re-examination of findings which were positive on the previous examination, although need not be limited to same. Reassessment is also indicated in the case of trauma or change in the clinical status of a patient.

Rating: Established

Evidence: E, L

Commentary

The term subluxation has a long history in the healing arts literature. It may be used differently outside of the chiropractic profession. The earliest non-chiropractic English definition is attributed to Randall Holme in 1668. Holme defined subluxation as "a dislocation or putting out of joynt"[5] In medical literature, subluxation often refers to an osseous disrelationship which is less than a dislocation.[6] However, B.J. Palmer, the developer of chiropractic, hypothesized that the "vertebral subluxation" was unique from the medical use of the term "subluxation" in that it also interfered with the transmission of neurological information independent of what has come to be recognized as the action potential. Since this component has yet to be identified in a quantitative sense, practitioners currently assess the presence and correction of vertebral subluxation through parameters which measure its other components.[7] These may include some type of vertebral biomechanical abnormality,[8-14] soft tissue insult of the spinal cord and/or associated structures[15-49] and some form of neurological dysfunction involving the synapse separate from the transmission of neurological information referred to by Palmer.[50-57]

As noted, chiropractic definitions of subluxation include a neurological component. In this regard, Lantz [58] stated "common to all concepts of subluxation are some form of kinesiologic[al...sic] dysfunction and some form of neurologic[al...sic] involvement." In a recently adopted position paper, The Association of Chiropractic Colleges accepted a definition of subluxation as follows: "A subluxation is a complex of functional and/or structural and/or pathological articular changes that compromise neural integrity and may influence organ system function and general health."[59] The case history and examination are means of acquiring information pertinent to the location and analysis of subluxation. This information is primarily used to characterize subluxation regarding its presence, location, duration, and type. Additionally, the information gained through analysis guides the practitioner to ascertain which chiropractic techniques best suit the patient to effect correction of the condition.

Data collected during the patient's initial consultation and examination, pertaining to the health history and presenting concerns, thus supports the decision-making process of the practitioner. This information, relayed by the practitioner to the patient, further serves to incorporate the patient into the decision-making process regarding chiropractic care.

Elements of the Examination

History

Important elements of the case history include previous and present social and occupational events revealed by the patient; unusual sensations, moods or actions relative to the patient, with dates of occurrence and duration; previous chiropractic and non-chiropractic intervention; and other factors. The case history usually includes the following:

1. Patient clinical profile.
    A. Age.
    B. Gender.
    C. Occupation.
    D. Other information germane to the presenting complaint, if any.
2. Primary reasons for seeking chiropractic care.
    A. Primary reason.
    B. Secondary reason.
    C. Other factors contributing to the primary and secondary reasons.
3. Chief complaint, if one exists. This may include onset and duration of symptoms as well as their subjective and objective characteristics, and location, as well as aggravating or relieving factors.
    A Trauma, by etiology, when possible.
    B. Chief complaint.
    C. Characteristics of chief complaint.
    D. Intensity/frequency/location, radiation/onset/duration.

     E.   Aggravating/arresting factors.

     F.   Previous interventions (including chiropractic care), treatments, medications, surgery.

     G.   Quality of pain, if present.

     H.   Sleeping position and sleep patterns.

4.   Family history.

     A.   Associated health problems of relatives.

     B.   Cause of parents' or siblings' death and age of death.

5.   Past health history.

     A.   Overall health status.

     B.   Previous illnesses.

     C.   Surgery.

     D.   Previous injury or trauma.

     E.   Medication and reactions.

     F.   Allergies.

     G.   Pregnancies and outcomes.

     H.   Substance abuse and outcomes.

6. Social and occupational history.

     A.   Level of education.

     B.   Job description.

     C.   Work schedule.

     D.   Recreational activities.

     E.   Lifestyle (hobbies, level of exercise, drug use, nature of diet).

     F.   Psychosocial and mental health.

Chiropractic Analysis

Complementing the case history is the necessity of conducting a thorough chiropractic analysis. This involves procedures which indicate the presence, location, and character of vertebral subluxation. Inherent in this process is the noting of unusual findings, both related and unrelated to vertebral subluxation. This information is useful in determining the safety and appropriateness of chiropractic care.

The analysis is based partly upon the recognition that vertebral subluxation may be asymptomatic, yet still exert various physiological effects. Thus, by assimilating information relative to certain body systems, the presence of vertebral subluxation may be inferred. Examination protocols have been developed by field practitioners and researchers.

Many of these protocols have been deemed acceptable by the various chiropractic educational institutions. This acceptance is expressed either through adding the protocols to the curriculum, or awarding continuing education credit to post-graduate seminars instructing these protocols, thus judging them to be sufficient in safety, efficacy, and validity to be included in clinical practice.

Manual palpation is a basic element of the chiropractic examination. This aspect of analysis includes palpation of the bony elements of the spine and includes assessment of the motion of the spine as a whole as well as the individual vertebral motion segments. Palpation of the numerous muscles which attach to and control the stability, posture, and motion of the spine is included. Static vertebral position is analyzed for abnormality. The chiropractor is additionally interested in locating areas of abnormal segmental motion to identify hypermobile segments and segments with decreased joint play (hypomobility). Palpation may also include evaluation of soft tissue compliance, tenderness, and asymmetric or hypertonic muscle contraction. The presence of vertebral subluxation may bring with it varying degrees of attendant edema, capsulitis, muscle splinting, and tenderness to digital palpation. There may be tenderness of the spinous processes upon percussion of these structures when vertebral subluxation is present.

Neurological components of the subluxation, postural distortions and other factors may bring deep and superficial myospasm to muscles of the spine, pelvis and extremities. Palpation may reveal myofascial trigger points which are associated with the articular dysfunctions accompanying vertebral subluxations. Muscular involvement may manifest as "taut and tender" fibers.

Visual inspection of the spine and paraspinal region may reveal areas of hypo- or hyperemia associated with vertebral subluxation. Observation of patient posture is an important element of chiropractic analysis.[60-62] Posture has far-reaching effects on physiology, biomechanics, psychology, and esthetics.[63] Proper body alignment relates to functional efficiency while poor structural alignment limits function. Changes in posture are considered in some chiropractic approaches as a measure of outcome.[64-69] Plain film radiographs, as well as other forms of imaging may provide information concerning the integrity of osseous and soft tissues as well as juxtapositional relationships. Other assessments such as leg length analysis,[70-94] palpatory and strength challenges[95-130] are also employed to assess states of muscular responses to neurological facilitation. Spinal distortions and resultant neurological interference may create postural or neurological reflex syndromes which result in a functional change in apparent leg length. This information is also combined with skin temperature assessments[131-138] and/or electromyography[139-167, 175-180] as well as technique-specific examination procedures to evaluate the integrity of the nervous system[181-182] Although clinical tradition supports the use of orthopedic and neurological tests in chiropractic practice, research to support the applicability of many of these tests to the assessment of vertebral subluxation is lacking or negative.[168-174] Orthopedic and neurological tests are indicated only when relevant to the assessment of vertebral subluxation, or when determining the safety and appropriateness of chiropractic care.

It is recognized that research will continue to evolve the most efficacious applications of assessment techniques described in this document. However, the literature is sufficiently supportive of their usefulness in regard to the chiropractic examination to warrant inclusion as components of the present recommendation.

The chiropractic examination may include, but not be limited to:

1. Clinical examination procedures.
   A. Palpation (static osseous and muscular, motion).
   B. Range of motion.
   C. Postural examination.
   D. Muscle strength testing.
   E. Orthopedic/neurological tests.
   F. Mental status examination procedures.
   G. Quality of life assessment instruments.
   H. Substance abuse and outcomes.
2. Imaging and instrumentation
   A. Plain film radiography.
   B. Videofluoroscopy.
   C. Computerized tomography.
   D. Magnetic resonance imaging.
   E. Range of motion.
   F. Thermography.
   G. Temperature reading instruments.
   H. Electromyography.
   I. Pressure algometry.

        J.   Nerve/function tests.
        K.   Electroencephalography.
    3. Review of systems.
        A.   Musculoskeletal.
        B.   Cardiovascular and respiratory.
        C.   Gastrointestinal.
        D.   Genitourinary.
        E.   Nervous system.
        F.   Eye, ear, nose and throat.
        G.   Endocrine.

Clinical Impression

An appropriate interpretation of case history and examination find-ings is essential in determining the appropriate application of chiropractic care within the overall needs of the patient. The clinical impression derived from patient information acquired through the examination process is ultimately translated into a plan of corrective care, including those elements which are contraindicated. The clinical impression serves to focus the practitioner on the patient's immediate and long-term needs. It is through this process that a clear picture is created regarding the patient's status relative to chiropractic care.

Initial Consultation

The initial consultation serves the purpose of determining how chi-ropractic care can benefit the patient. It is during this interchange that the practitioner presents and discusses examination findings with the patient. Additionally, during the initial consultation, the practitioner should take the opportunity to present his/her practice objectives and terms of accep-tance. The terms of acceptance provides the patient with information regarding the objectives, responsibilities and limitations of the care to be provided by the practitioner. This reciprocal acknowledgment allows both practitioner and patient to proceed into the plan of care with well-defined expectations.

While not limited to the following, it is suggested that the initial con-sultation include the following parameters:

1. Description of chiropractic: Chiropractic is a primary contact health care profession receiving patients without necessity of referral from other health care providers. Traditionally, chiropractic focuses on the

anatomy of the spine and its immediate articulations, the existence and nature of vertebral subluxation, and a scope of practice which encompasses the correction of vertebral subluxation, as well as educating and advising patients concerning this condition, and its impact on general health.

2. Professional responsibility: To assess the propriety of applying methods of analysis and vertebral subluxation correction to patients; to recognize and deal appropriately with emergency situations; and to report to the patient any nonchiropractic findings discovered during the course of the examination, making referral to other health professionals for care or for evaluation of conditions outside the scope of chiropractic practice. Such referral does not obviate the responsibility of the chiropractor for providing appropriate chiropractic care.

3. Practice objective: The professional practice objective of the chiropractor is to correct or stabilize the vertebral subluxation in a safe and effective manner. The correction of vertebral subluxation is not considered a specific cure or treatment for any specific medical disease or symptom. Rather, it is applicable to any patient exhibiting vertebral subluxation, regardless of the presence or absence of symptoms and diseases.

2   Instrumentation

RECOMMENDATION

Instrumentation is indicated for the qualitative and/or quantitative assessment of the biomechanical and physiological components of vertebral subluxation. When using instrumentation, baseline values should be determined prior to the initiation of care.

Rating: Established
Evidence: E, L

Commentary

The chiropractor uses a variety of procedures to assess the vertebral subluxation. These methods may include history taking, physical examination, imaging procedures and instrumentation. Through information gained from research and personal experience, the chiropractor generally assigns a personal value to each procedure in a particular clinical circumstance. The intent of this chapter is to describe clinical applications for the various instruments that may be used by chiropractors in examining their patients for evidence of vertebral subluxation.

Definition of instrumentation: The use of any tool or device used to obtain objective data, which can be recorded in a reproducible manner, about the condition of the patient relative to vertebral subluxation. Such instrumentation as that described below may provide information concerning the biomechanical and/or neurological aspects of vertebral subluxation.

POSTURAL ANALYSIS

Sub-Recommendation

Postural analysis using plumb line devices, computerized and non-computerized instruments may be used to evaluate changes in posture associated with vertebral subluxation.

Rating: Established
Evidence: E, L

Posture analysis is recommended for determining postural aberrations associated with vertebral subluxation. The findings of such examinations should be recorded in the patient record. In order to encourage standardization of reporting, it is suggested that findings be recorded in a form consistent with manufacturers' recommendations.

Posture analysis may include the use of such devices as the plumb line, scoliometer and posturometer.[1-8] Posture is often analyzed by x-ray methods[9-13] simply by visualizing the patient and making determinations based on that visualization. The procedure is often enhanced by a plumb line and other vertical and horizontal lines.

BILATERAL AND FOUR-QUADRANT WEIGHT SCALES

Sub-Recommendation

Bilateral and four-quadrant weight scales may be used to determine the weight distribution asymmetries indicative of spinal abnormalities.

Rating: Established
Evidence: E, L

Unequal weight distribution has been shown to be indicative of spinal abnormalities.[14-18] Weight scales are a simple and effective means to determine weight distribution asymmetries.

MOIRÉ CONTOUROGRAPHY

Sub-Recommendation

Moiré contourography may be used to provide a photographic record of changes in body contour associated with vertebral subluxation.
Rating: Established
Evidence: E, L

Moiré contourography is a photographic technique which yields information regarding body contours and their variations for the purpose of evaluating structural abnormality. It is useful to the chiropractor because body surface asymmetries may be indicative of the presence of vertebral subluxation.[19-33]

INCLINOMETRY

Inclinometry may be used as a means of measuring motion against a constant vertical component of gravity as a reference. Changes in ranges of spinal motion may be associated with vertebral subluxation.
Rating: Established
Evidence: E, L

Mechanical, electronic and fluid-filled inclinometers are available.[34-38] Inclinometer measurements have been thoroughly studied regarding their ability to measure complex motions of the spine.[39-49] Inclinometers are considered superior to goniometers for assessing spinal motion.[50] Inclinometers have been shown to be accurate within 10% of those obtained by radiographic evaluation.[51] Achieving acceptable reliability is dependent upon use of standardized procedures.

GONIOMETRY

Sub-Recommendation

Goniometry, computer associated or not, may be used to measure

joint motion. Inclinometry is superior to goniometry when standardized procedures are employed.

Rating: Established

Evidence: E, L

A goniometer is a protractor that may be held in the proximity of the area being measured to provide a means by which to determine degrees of motion.[35] Although goniometry is common, a wide range of variance has been reported, [56-59] expressing up to 10°-15° error.[60, 61]

ALGOMETRY

Sub-Recommendation

Algometry may be used to measure pressure-pain threshold. Changes in sensory function associated with vertebral subluxation may produce changes in pressure-pain thresholds.

Rating: Established

Evidence: E, L

A pressure-pain threshold meter yields a measurement of when a patient feels a change from pressure to tenderness as the device produces mechanical irritation of deep somatic structures. Pressure-pain-threshold measurements produce acceptable levels of reliability.[62-66, 142-145] Algometry has been shown to be very useful in measuring changes in paraspinal tissue tenderness as the thresholds are symmetrical.[145] This renders the procedure applicable to chiropractic analysis.

CURRENT PERCEPTION THRESHOLD (CPT) TESTING

Sub-Recommendation

Current perception threshold devices may be used for the quantitative assessment of sensory nerve function. Alterations in sensory nerve function may be associated with vertebral subluxation.

Rating: Established

Evidence: E, L

The current perception threshold device is a variable voltage constant current sine wave stimulator proposed as a simple noninvasive and quantitative measure of peripheral nerve function.[67-71, 137-141] One type of current perception threshold instrument, the neurometer, has been shown to be appropriate for rapid screening for neural dysfunction.[69]

ELECTROENCEPHALOGRAPHY (EEG)
Sub-Recommendation

Electroencephalographic techniques including brain mapping and spectral analysis, may be used to assess the effects of vertebral subluxation and chiropractic adjustment associated with brain function.
Rating: Established
Evidence: E, L

Standard EEG and computerized EEG techniques, including spectral analysis and brain mapping, have been shown to change following chiropractic adjustments or manipulation.[72, 161, 204] Such procedures may be useful in evaluating possible effects of chiropractic care on brain function.

SOMATOSENSORY EVOKED POTENTIALS (SSEP)
Sub-Recommendation

Somatosensory evoked potentials may be used for localizing neurological dysfunction associated with vertebral subluxations.
Rating: Established
Evidence: E, L

Somatosensory and dermatomal evoked potentials are used for localizing neurological abnormalities in the peripheral and central conducting pathways. These findings are useful as objective indicators of the level or levels of involvement.[73-86, 154] One study reported that improved nerve root function was observed in subjects who received a high-velocity chiropractic thrust; similar changes were not observed in controls.[73]

SKIN TEMPERATURE INSTRUMENTATION
Sub-Recommendation

Temperature reading devices employing thermocouples, infrared thermometry, or thermography (liquid crystal, telethermography, multiple IR detector, etc.) may be used to detect temperature changes in

spinal and paraspinal tissues related to vertebral subluxation.
Rating: Established
Evidence: E, L

The measurement of paraspinal cutaneous thermal asymmetries and other measurements of anomalies have been shown to be a mode of sympathetic nervous system assessment, [88, 90, 91, 93-95, 97-103, 160] which may be used as one indicator of vertebral subluxation. Demonstrable changes in thermal patterns have been observed following chiropractic adjustment.[19, 92] Thermocouple instruments have been shown to demonstrate an acceptable level of reliability and clinical utility applicable to the assessment of vertebral subluxation related temperature changes.[87, 89, 96, 104] Normative data have been collected concerning the degree of thermal asymmetry in the human body in healthy subjects.[105] These values may serve as one standard in the assessment of sympathetic nerve function and the degree of asymmetry as a quantifiable indicator of possible dysfunction.[106]

SURFACE ELECTROMYOGRAPHY

Sub-Recommendation

Surface electrode electromyography, using hand-held electrodes, or affixed electrodes, may be used for recording changes in the electrical activity of muscles associated with vertebral subluxations.
Rating: Established
Evidence: E, L, C

Surface electromyographic techniques using both hand-held electrodes and affixed electrodes have demonstrated an acceptable level of reliability for general clinical usage.[107-112, 114-121, 129-136, 159] Other studies have demonstrated that significant changes in muscle electrical activity occur following adjustment or spinal manipulation.[111, 113, 126, 136] Protocols and normative data for paraspinal EMG scanning in chiropractic practice have been published.[122-125, 127-128] Surface EMG techniques may be used to assess changes in paraspinal muscle activity associated with vertebral subluxation and chiropractic adjustment.

MUSCLE STRENGTH TESTING

Sub-Recommendation

Muscle strength testing may be used to determine bilateral differ-

ences or other differences in patient resistance. These differences may be characterized by the experienced examiner based on various technologies. Manual, mechanized and computerized muscle testing may be used to determine changes in the strength and other characteristics of muscles. These changes may be a result of alterations of function at various levels of the neuromuscular system and/or any other system related to the patient. Such changes may be associated with vertebral subluxation.

Rating: Established

Evidence: E, L

Muscle testing as a means of evaluation and diagnosis of patients within chiropractic as well as other disciplines, is well documented.[146-153, 155-158, 163-177] Muscle testing techniques may be used to assess the effect of vertebral subluxation on various aspects of muscle strength. Research has shown manual muscle testing to be sufficiently reliable for clinical practice. [148, 149, 153, 156, 169, 170, 171, 175] Studies concerning manual muscle testing have also demonstrated electromyographic differences associated with various muscle weaknesses, and differences in somatosensory evoked potentials associated with weak versus strong muscles.[146, 147] Other studies have demonstrated the clinical utility and reliability of hand-held muscle strength testing devices.[151, 152, 157, 172]

QUESTIONNAIRES
Sub-Recommendation

Questionnaires may be used in the assessment of the performance of activities of daily living, pain perception, patient satisfaction, general health outcomes, patient perception outcomes, mental health outcomes, and overall quality of life, throughout a course of chiropractic care. Questionnaires provide important information, but should not be used as a substitute for physical indicators of the presence and character of vertebral subluxations.

Rating: Established

Evidence: E, L

There are a variety of questionnaires of demonstrated reliability and validity which may be used to document outcomes,[178-203] including pain and symptoms, although these are not necessary correlates of vertebral subluxation. However, correction of vertebral subluxation and reduction of the abnormal spinal and general functions associated with it may be accompanied by reduction or elimination of pain and symptoms. It must be emphasized that the clinical objective of chiropractic care is the correction of vertebral subluxations. No questionnaires exist which assess the presence or correction of vertebral subluxation. Therefore, it is inappropriate to employ questionnaires to determine the need for chiropractic care, but questionnaires are appropriate as one aspect of monitoring patient progress and the effectiveness of subluxation-based care.

3   Radiographic and Other Imaging

RECOMMENDATION

Diagnostic imaging procedures may be utilized to characterize the biomechanical manisfestations of vertebral subluxation, and to determine the presence of conditions which affect the safety and appropriateness of chiropractic care.

Sub-Recommendation

Plain film radiography is indicated: to provide information concerning the structural integrity of the spine, skull and pelvis; the misalignment component of the vertebral subluxation; the foraminal alteration component of the vertebral subluxation; and the postural status of the spinal column. Imaging procedures, including post-adjustment radiography, should be performed only when clinically necessary. It is common for lines of mensuration to be drawn on radiographs to assess subluxation and alignment. These procedures may be done by hand, or the chiropractor may utilize computerized radiographic digitization procedures.

Rating: Established
Evidence: E, L

Commentary

In considering the use of imaging methods employing ionizing radiation as a component of patient assessment, the clinician should determine if the methods of subluxation correction, patient safety, and management require the use of such procedures. The patient should be asked about any conditions which may contraindicate certain imaging procedures.

Reliability studies of several systems of biomechanical analysis, including radiographic marking systems, have been published. Imaging is a necessary component of a number of different chiropractic analyses. The preponderance of evidence supports the reliability of these procedures when properly performed.[1-8, 12, 15-27, 29-32, 36-39, 42-61, 64-68, 70-79, 153]

Moreover, radiographic imaging has revealed statistically significant changes in the direction of atlas positioning following chiropractic adjustment(s).[14, 28, 33-35, 146-148] The effect of chiropractic care on lateral curvature of the cervical spine has been investigated, with significant changes in the cervical curve noted in patients receiving chiropractic care.[9, 62, 63, 69, 149-152, 156-158]

Sub-Recommendation

Imaging procedures employing ionizing radiation should be performed consistent with the principles of obtaining films of high quality with minimal radiation. This may include the use of gonad shielding, compensating filters, and appropriate film-screen combinations.

Rating: Established

Evidence: E, L

A number of dosimetry studies using supplemental filtration and single-speed screens have revealed that in the case of 14 x 36 inch AP full-spine radiographs, the radiation levels were less than sectional films of like-sized subjects. Shielding of radiosensitive structures may be used when it does not obliterate structures of clinical interest. Such shielding results in a reduction of radiation exposure.[10, 11, 13, 160]

Conclusion

The judicious use of spinographic techniques can be valuable in characterizing aspects of the biomechanical manifestations of vertebral subluxation.[146, 154, 155, 187-193] The use of post-adjustment radiographs may also assist the chiropractor in determining effects of chiropractic adjustments on the spine when other less hazardous examination techniques cannot reveal the desired information.

VIDEOFLUOROSCOPY

Sub-Recommendation

Videofluoroscopy may be employed to provide motion views of the spine when abnormal motion patterns are clinically suspected. Videofluoroscopy may be valuable in detecting and characterizing spinal kinesiopathology associated with vertebral subluxation.

Rating: Established

Evidence: E, L

Commentary

A videofluoroscopic system consists of an x-ray generator capable of operating at low (1/4 to 5) milliamperage settings, an x-ray tube assembly, an image intensifier tube, a television camera, a VCR, and a monitor. The heart of the system is the image intensifier tube. This tube permits imaging at very low radiation levels. It is used instead of intensifying screens and film as a image receptor.

The role of videofluoroscopy in the evaluation of abnormalities of spinal motion has been discussed in textbooks, medical journals, and chiropractic publications.[19, 20, 23, 80-83, 140, 145, 163, 164, 168-170, 172-179, 186, 220] Studies have appeared in the literature comparing the diagnostic yield of fluoroscopic studies versus plain films, as well as reporting abnormalities detected by fluoroscopy which could not be assessed using plain films.[161, 165-167, 171, 180, 183-185]

Reliability has been addressed in a number of studies.[162, 181, 182, 214] Additionally, in a study evaluating the interexaminer reliability of fluoroscopic detection of fixation in the mid-cervical spine, two examiners reviewed 50 videotapes of fluoroscopic examinations of the cervical spine. The examiners achieved 84 percent agreement for the presence of fixation, 96 percent agreement for the absence of fixation, and 93 percent total agreement. The Kappa value was .80 (p<.001). The authors concluded, "The current data indicate that VF determination of fixation in the cervical spine is a reliable procedure." [181, 214]

Conclusion

Observational and case studies support the use of videofluoroscopy to evaluate vertebral motion when this information cannot be obtained by other means.

Sub-Recommendation

Magnetic Resonance Imaging (MRI)

MR imaging may be employed to assess suspected neoplastic, infectious and degenerative conditions of the spine and related tissues as well as the stages of subluxation degeneration. Its use is generally restricted to instances where the desired information cannot be obtained by less costly procedures.

Rating: Established
Evidence: E, L

Commentary

Magnetic resonance imaging enables clinicians to obtain clear images of the human body without ionizing radiation.

Literature supports the use of MR imaging for the detection and characterization of numerous manifestations associated with subluxation degeneration.[84-107, 141-143, 194-198, 212] These studies cover a spectrum of phenomena, including:

1. Osseous malalignment
2. Intervertebral disc desiccation and degeneration
3. Osteophytosis
4. Corrugation/hypertrophy of the ligamentum flava
5. Spinal canal stenosis
6. Foraminal stenosis
7. Disc herniation and disc bulging
8. Facet asymmetry
9. Facet degeneration
10. Altered cerebrospinal fluid dynamics
11. Cord compression
12. Gliosis and myelomalacia
13. Spinal cord atrophy

Conclusion

MRI may be employed to disclose manifestations of vertebral subluxation when this information cannot be obtained by more cost-effective means. MRI is also appropriate for evaluating patients with clinical evidence of conditions which may affect the safety and appropriateness of chiropractic procedures.

Sub-Recommendation

Computed Tomography (CT)

CT imaging may be employed to assess osseous and soft tissue pathology in the spine and contiguous tissues. Its use is generally restricted to instances where the desired information cannot be obtained by less costly procedures.

Rating: Established
Evidence: E, L

Commentary

Computed tomography (also referred to as CT or CAT scanning) is an imaging technique which produces axial (cross sectional) images of body structures using x-radiation. Computer reconstruction methods may be used to depict other planes.

Manifestations of subluxation degeneration which may be demonstrated by CT scanning include disc lesions, spinal canal stenosis due to infolding of the ligamentum flava, osteophytosis, and bony sclerosis.[108-139, 144, 199-201, 210, 211, 213, 220] In addition, CT may be used to evaluate developmental variance and pathologies which could affect the chiropractic management of a case.

Conclusion

CT may be employed to disclose manifestations of vertebral subluxation when this information cannot be obtained by more cost-effective means. CT is also appropriate for evaluating patients with clinical evidence of conditions which may affect the safety and appropriateness of chiropractic procedures, particularly fractures, degenerative changes, and osseous pathology.

Sub-Recommendation

Spinal Ultrasonography

Spinal ultrasonography may be used to evaluate the size of the spinal canal, and to detect pathology in the soft tissues surrounding the spine. Its applications in the assessment of the facet inflammation and nerve root inflammation remain investigational at this time.

Ratings: Established for determining spinal canal size.

Investigational for facet and nerve root inflammation.

Evidence: E, L

Commentary

Sonographic imaging is a technique which utilizes echoes from ultrasonic waves to produce an image on a cathode ray tube.

Sonographic techniques have been employed to measure the lumbar canal, as well as determining focal stenosis and disc disease.[202-209, 221, 222]

A small study compared sonographic results in patients with back pain previously examined by MRI, x-ray and standard orthopedic examination. The study concluded that the correlation with MRI, x-ray, orthopedic and neurologic examination was approximately 90 percent.[207]

Conclusion

The low cost, availability, ease of application, and noninvasive nature of sonographic imaging make it an attractive addition to the chiropractor's armamentarium. Furthermore, it has the potential to image various components of the vertebral subluxation. However, caution must be exercised in evaluating the claims of promoters of sonographic equipment, particularly those relating to the assessment of nerve root inflammation or facet joint disease. Further research toward the establishment of chiropractic protocols should be undertaken to explore the clinical utility of spinal sonography in chiropractic practice.

Sub-Recommendation

Radioisotope Scanning (Nuclear Medicine Studies)

Radioisotope scans performed by qualified medical personnel may be used by a chiropractor to determine the extent and distribution of pathological processes which may affect the safety and appropriateness of chiropractic care when this information cannot be obtained by less invasive means.

Rating: Established
Evidence: E, L

Commentary

In this procedure, bone-seeking radioisotopes are injected, and an image is produced demonstrating the degree of uptake of the radioisotopes. The examination is sensitive to regional changes in osseous metabolism, but is not specific. Abnormal bone scans may be due to metastasis, infection, fracture, osteoblastic activity or other pathology.[215-219] No studies or case reports were found linking abnormal bone scans with vertebral subluxation. Bone scans may have limited value in determining the safety and appropriateness of chiropractic procedures.

Conclusion

Radioisotope scans have a limited role in chiropractic practice. Bone scans are a sensitive, but nonspecific indicator of abnormal metabolic activity in bone.

4   Clinical Impression and Assessment

RECOMMENDATION

Practitioners should develop a method of patient assessment which includes a sufficient diversity of findings to support the clinical impression as related to vertebral subluxation.(1-24) In this regard, it is considered inappropriate to render an opinion regarding the appropriateness of chiropractic care without a chiropractic assessment, including a physical examination of the patient by a licensed chiropractor. When management of patient care is carried out in the collaborative setting, the chiropractor, as a primary contact health care provider, is the only professional qualified to determine the appropriateness of chiropractic care. The unique role of the chiropractor is separate from other health disciplines,(25-35) and should be clarified for both the patient and other practitioners. The patient assessment, specific to the technique practiced by the chiropractor, should minimally include a biomechanical and neurophysiological component. It is inappropriate to make a retrospective determination of the clinical need for care rendered prior to the assessment.

Rating: Established
Evidence: E, L

Commentary

The procedures employed in the chiropractic assessment may include some or all of, but are not limited to the following:

Physical examination:

Palpation (static osseous, static muscle, motion).
Range of motion.
Postural examination
Comparative leg length (static, flexed, cervical syndrome).
Manual muscle tests.
Nerve function tests.
Mental status examination and psychosocial assessment.

Instrumentation examination:
Range of motion.
Thermography.
Temperature reading instruments.
Muscle testing.
Electromyography.
Pressure algometry.
Nerve-function tests.
Electroencephalography and brain mapping.
Bilateral and four quadrant weight scales.

Imaging examination:
Spinography.
Videofluoroscopy.
Computerized tomography.

Magnetic resonance imaging.

Following the determination of a clinical impression, the patient should be made aware of the findings and consent to the proposed plan of care.

Literature support for the use of these technologies may be found in the chapters on chiropractic examination, instrumentation and diagnostic imaging (Chapters 1, 2, 3).

5 Reassessment and Outcomes Assessment

RECOMMENDATION

Determination of the patient's progress must be made on a per-visit and periodic basis. This process provides quantitative and qualitative information regarding the patient's progress which is utilized to determine the frequency and duration of chiropractic care. Per-visit reassessment should include at least one analytical procedure previously used. This chosen testing procedure should be performed each time the patient receives chiropractic care.

Concomitant with this process, the effectiveness of patient care may also be monitored through the development of an outcomes assessment plan. Such a plan may utilize data from the patient examination, assessment and reassessment procedures. Patient-reported quality of life instruments, mental health surveys, and general health surveys are encouraged as part of the outcomes assessment plan. The analysis of data from these sources may be used to change or support continuation of a particular regimen of patient care and/or change or continue the operational procedures of the practice.

Rating: Established

Evidence: E, L

Commentary

The reassessment provides information to determine the necessity of an adjustment on a per-visit basis. Partial reassessment involves duplica-

127

tion of two or more preceding positive analytical procedures. Full reassessment involves duplication of three or more preceding positive analytical procedures. Any additional or complementary analytical procedures should be performed as indicated by the patient's clinical status. The frequency of partial and full reassessments should be at the discretion of the practitioner, consistent with the objectives of the plan of care.

A substantial body of literature attests to the methods and significance of measuring outcomes.[1-100] For the practicing chiropractor the implication is that regular evaluations of practice and procedures provides a form of quality control. Outcomes assessments can alert the practitioner to problems with, as well as reinforce, aspects of practice which might otherwise be overlooked. In addition, on-going evaluation provides information about the clinical value of care to both patients and third-party providers. It is important to point out that there is no one "ideal" way to assess outcomes. While the responsibility to conduct this type of assessment rests with the chiropractor, so does the choice of how it is to be implemented.

6   Modes of Adjustive Care

RECOMMENDATION

Adjusting procedures should be selected which are determined by the practitioner to be safe and effective for the individual patient. No mode of care should be used which has been demonstrated by critical scientific study and field experience to be unsafe or ineffective in the correction of vertebral subluxation.

Rating: Established

Evidence: E, L

Commentary

This chapter is concerned with the modes of adjustive care (techniques) associated with the correction of vertebral subluxation. The literature reveals many articles on adjusting modes. These articles include technique descriptions, various applications of techniques, and reliability studies usually assessing inter- and intra-examiner reliability. A number of review articles provide discussion of the modes of care. Available research data has been complemented with professional opinion, derived from two separate forums of chiropractic experts' The International Straight Chiropractic Consensus Conference, Chandler, Arizona (1992) and the Council on Chiropractic Practice Symposium on Chiropractic Techniques, Phoenix, Arizona, (1996), both of which served to validate procedures by common knowledge and usage.

The intent of this chapter is not to include nor exclude any particular technique, but rather to provide a guideline, drawing upon the commonality of various techniques, which contributes to the chiropractic objective of correcting vertebral subluxation. Any technique which does not espouse the correction of subluxation would be considered outside the scope of the Guideline.

A list of descriptive terms and definitions related to chiropractic adjustive care as commonly practiced follows:

Adjustment: The correction of a vertebral subluxation.

Adjustic Thrust: The specific application of force to facilitate the correction of vertebral subluxation.

Adjusting Instruments: Fixed or hand-held mechanical instruments used to deliver a specific, controlled thrust to correct a vertebral subluxation.

Amplitude: Magnitude; greatness of size or depth.

Blocking Technique: The use of mechanical leverage, achieved through positioning of the spine or related structures, to facilitate the correction of vertebral subluxation.

Cleavage: The movement of one vertebra between two other vertebrae.

Concussion: An adjustic thrust produced by arrested momentum. Momentum is the result of weight (mass) in motion and also of speed. An adjustic concussion depends more on speed than mass.

High Velocity Thrust with Recoil: A controlled thrust delivered such that the time of impact with the vertebra coincides with the chiropractor's contact recoil, thus setting the vertebra in a specific directional motion.

Impulse: A sudden force directionally applied to correct a malpositioned joint.

Low Velocity Thrust with Recoil: A controlled thrust administered at low speed with a sudden pull-off by the practitioner, setting the segment in motion.

Low Velocity Thrust without Recoil: A controlled thrust administered at low speed coupled with a sustained contact on the segment adjusted.

Low Velocity Vectored Force without Recoil: A short or long duration (usually ranging from 1 to 20 seconds) contact with the segment being adjusted, with or without a graduation of force.

Manually Assisted Mechanical Thrust: A manually delivered specific thrust enhanced by a moving mechanism built into the adjusting table.

Manipulation: The taking of a joint past its passive range of motion into the paraphysiological space but not past the anatomic limit, accompanied by articular cavitation (Kirkaldy-Willis). It is not synonymous with chiropractic adjustment, which is applied to correct vertebral subluxation.

Multiple Impulse: Impulses delivered in rapid succession.

Recoil: The bouncing or springing back of an object when it strikes another object.

Tone: The normal degree of nerve tension.

Thrust: The act of putting a bony segment in motion using a directional force.

Toggle: A mechanical principle wherein two levers are hinged at an elbow giving mechanical advantage. Combinations of toggles may be used to multiply or strengthen mechanical advantage.

Toggle Recoil with Torque: A method of using the toggle with rotation (twist) as the toggle straightens, causing the adjusting contact to travel in a spiral path.

Torque: A rotational or twisting vector applied when adjusting certain vertebral subluxations.

Velocity: The speed with which a thrust is delivered.

Conclusion

Considerable evidence substantiates the adjustment being administered for the purpose of correction of vertebral subluxation.[1-11] Studies regarding the different modes[4, 12-86] compare low force methods to those employing a high velocity thrust without recoil, and low velocity vectored force without recoil, high velocity thrust with recoil, low velocity thrust with and without recoil, manually and mechanically assisted thrusts, blocking techniques, and sustained force. These studies are often presented in the context of effects on various physical and physiological parameters.

Although providing useful information, the majority of these studies are limited by uncontrolled variables and lack of statistical power. They do, however, demonstrate that the application of various modes of adjustive care is accompanied by measurable changes in physical and physiological phenomena. The importance of this information, in terms of its linkage to processes used by the body in the correction of subluxation, will be assessed through continued research.

These guidelines consider[86] the modes of adjustive care in common usage, which adhere to one or more of the descriptive terms presented in this chapter, as appropriate for correction of subluxation. However, studies regarding their theoretical basis and efficacy are often conducted by advocates of (those practicing or instructing) the respective techniques. While the information attained in the numerous investigations is not in question, since many of the studies have not passed the scrutiny of peer and editorial review, it is suggested that the advocates of particular modes of adjustive care encourage research by chiropractic colleges, independent universities and other facilities to extend the level of credibility already achieved.

Continuing research and reliability studies are necessary to better understand and refine the underlying mechanisms of action common to the various modes of adjustive care. In addition, it is suggested that more observational and patient self-reporting studies be conducted which deal with quality of life assessments and overall "wellness," to demonstrate the pattern of health benefits which heretofore have been the purview of the patient and the practitioner. A conference sponsored by U.S. Department of Health and Human Services, Public Health Service Agency for Health Care Policy and Research, proposed many different approaches for studying the effects of treatments for which there is no direct evidence of health outcomes.[87]

The CCP recognizes that many subluxation-based chiropractors do not adhere, in totality, to the current hypothetical model thus far described. These practitioners consider two additional components. One is interference with the transmission of nonsynaptic neurological information which is homologous to the Palmer concept of mental impulse. The other limits the misalignment component of the subluxation to the vertebrae and their immediate articulations. While these practitioners may adhere to some concepts of other subluxation models, their practice objectives are based on correction of the vertebral subluxation as proposed by Palmer, which has recently been elaborated by Boone and Dobson.[88-90]

7 Duration of Care for Correction of Vertebral Subluxation

RECOMMENDATION

Since the duration of care for correction of vertebral subluxation is patient specific, frequency of visits should be based upon the reduction and eventual resolution of indicators of vertebral subluxation. Since neither the scientific nor clinical literature provides any compelling evidence that substantiates or correlates any specific time period for the correction of vertebral subluxation, this recommendation has several components which are expressed as follows:

a) Based on the variety of assessments utilized in the chiropractic profession, the quantity of indicators may vary, thus affecting the periodicity of their appearance and disappearance, which is tantamount to correction of vertebral subluxation.

b) Vertebral subluxation, not being a singular episodic event such as a strain or sprain, may be corrected but reappear, which necessitates careful monitoring and results in a wide variation in the number of adjustments required to affect a longer-term correction.

c) Based on the integrity of the spine in terms of degree and extent of degeneration, the frequency of assessments, and the necessity for corrective adjustments, may vary considerably.

d) Because the duration of care is being considered relative to the correction of vertebral subluxation, it is independent of clinical manifestations of specific dysfunctions, diseases, or syndromes. Treatment protocols and duration of care for these conditions are addressed in other guidelines, which may be appropriate for any practitioner whose clinical interests include alleviation of such conditions.

Rating: Established

Evidence: E, L

Commentary

Attempts have been made to identify an appropriate number and frequency of chiropractic visits based on type of condition and degree of severity.[1-24] Unfortunately, these recommendations are based merely on consensus, and research to support these recommendations is lacking. Moreover, little to no delineation has been made in the duration of care literature base between care for specific symptomatic profiles such as low-back pain, and long-term subluxation-specific care.

Two studies were found which addressed quality of life issues in patients under chiropractic care. One large, well-designed retrospective study assessing patient reported quality of life found no clinical end point where improvement reached a plateau.[25] A second study involved a detailed examination of a database collected during a randomized clinical trial testing the effectiveness of a comprehensive geriatric assessment program. It was reported that compared to non-chiropractic patients, chiropractic patients in this population were less likely to have been hospitalized, less likely to have used a nursing home, more likely to report a better health status, more likely to exercise vigorously, and more likely to be mobile in the community. Furthermore, they were less likely to use prescription drugs.[26]

It is the position of the Guideline Panel that individual differences in each patient and the unique circumstances of each clinical encounter preclude the formulation of "cookbook" recommendations for frequency and duration of care.

The appropriateness of chiropractic care should be determined by objective indicators of vertebral subluxation.

8   Chiropractic Care of Children

RECOMMENDATION

Since vertebral subluxation may affect individuals at any age, chiropractic care may be indicated at any time after birth. As with any age group, however, care must be taken to select adjustment methods most appropriate to the patient's stage of development and overall spinal integrity. Parental education by the subluxation-centered chiropractor

133

concerning the importance of evaluating children for the presence of vertebral subluxation is encouraged.

Rating: Established

Evidence: E, L

Commentary

Schneier and Burns[1] published the results of a blinded study describing the relationship of atlanto-occipital hypermobility to sudden infant death syndrome (SIDS). These authors described the phenomenon of "atlas inversion" where the posterior arch of C-1 enters the foramen magnum. They further stated, "Relative measurements suggested that a correlation existed between instability in the atlanto-occipital articulation and sudden infant death syndrome." Instability is a manifestation of vertebral subluxation.

These findings corroborate those of Gilles, Bina and Sotrel in their paper, "Infantile atlanto-occipital instability."[2] These investigators studied 17 infant cadavers. Eleven were SIDS cases and six were non-SIDS cases. Ten of the 17 cases demonstrated atlas inversion, and all ten cases were in the SIDS group. These authors also suggested that atlanto-occipital instability may be a factor in other conditions. They stated, "At this early stage in the development of our notions about the potential contribution of atlanto-occipital instability to deaths in infants, it is very difficult to assess the role of this proposed mechanism in the death of an infant with a conventional disease. Thus, one might anticipate that the 'controls' will be contaminated by children who had a conventional disease, but whose death was, in fact, caused by this mechanism."

Towbin[3] addressed the clinical significance of spinal cord and brain stem injury at birth, noting that such damage is often latent and undiagnosed. According to Towbin, "Death of the fetus may occur during delivery or, with respiratory function depressed, a short period after birth. Infants who survive the initial effects may be left with severe nervous system defects. In some, the neurologic sequellae are attributable directly to the primary lesion in the cord or brain stem; in others, secondary cerebral damage results, a consequence of the imposed period of hypoxia at birth." Chesire[4] described three cases of traumatic myelopathy in children without demonstrable vertebral trauma. In this paper, the classical mechanism of trauma is said to be hyperextension of the cervical spine in a difficult breech delivery. Although tetraplegia may result, the x-rays are described as "usually normal." Complicated deliveries represent a higher risk to the child of suffering spinal cord damage during the birth process. High cervical spinal cord injury in neonates is a specific complication of forceps rotation. The vacuum extractor exerts considerable traction force. Fetal skull fracture can result, and its true incidence may be higher than expected, considering that few neonates with normal neurologic behavior undergo skull x-ray.[5-7] Byers[8] published an excellent review paper addressing spinal cord damage during the birth process. Traction and rotational stresses applied to the spinal axis were listed as causes of spinal cord injury during birth.

The vagus nerve is involved in mechanisms associated with control of tidal volume, breathing rate, and respiratory reflexes. Sachis et al.[9] performed histological examinations of the vagus nerve in infants who died of SIDS and those who died of other conditions. Significant differences were noted between the two groups. Several hypotheses were proposed by authors to explain the data, including damage to the vagus nerve resulting in delayed development.

Gutman[10] described how "relational disturbance" between occiput and atlas can lead to "blocked atlantal nerve syndrome" in children and adults. The author listed a variety of conditions which appear clinically related to this syndrome. Although SIDS was not discussed as an entity, the author stated that a brain stem component is a part of this syndrome. It was concluded that for those affected, "manual treatment" by a qualified practitioner is appropriate.

In her paper "Physical stresses of childhood that could lead to need for chiropractic care," presented at the first National Conference on Chiropractic and Pediatrics, McMullen[11] stated, "Any condition that arises to change the normal birth process… frequently results in subluxation at the level of greatest stress. Severe subluxation resulting in nerve damage may be clinically obvious at birth (e.g., Bell's, Erb's and Klumpke's palsies), however, more frequently the trauma remains subclinical with symptoms arising at a later time. These symptoms include, but are not limited to, irritability, colic, failure-to-thrive syndromes, and those syndromes associated with lowered immune responses. These subluxations should be analyzed and corrected as soon as possible after birth to prevent these associated conditions."

Bonci and Wynne[12] and Stiga[13] published papers discussing the relationship between chiropractic theory and SIDS etiology. Banks et al.[14]

stated "Functional disturbances in the brainstem and cervical spinal cord areas related to the neurophysiology of respiration may contribute the clinical factors associated with sudden infant death syndrome... Any process, whether genetic, biochemical, biomechanical or traumatic, that alters normal development of the respiratory control centers related to spinal constriction and compression following birth trauma may be contributory to sudden infant death syndrome."

Other traumatic events of childhood may produce vertebral subluxations. Orenstein et al.[15] did a retrospective chart review involving 73 children who presented at a children's hospital with cervical spine injuries. Sixty-seven percent of these injuries were traffic related resulting from motor-vehicle crashes. The injured children were passengers in an automobile, pedestrians, or bicyclists. The mean age of the patients surveyed was 8.6 years, with bimodal peaks at 2 to 4 and 12 to 15 years. The authors noted that younger children sustained more severe injuries than older children. Distraction and subluxation injuries were the most common injuries in children aged 8 years and younger. Fractures were more common in older children.

Glass et al.[16] evaluated 35 children with lumbar spine injuries following blunt trauma. Thirty-one of these children were injured in motor-vehicle crashes. Abnormalities noted on plain radiographs and CT scans included subluxation, distraction, and fracture alone or in combination. The authors stated, "Children involved in motor-vehicle crashes are at a high risk for lumbar spine injuries... Lumbar spine radiographs are necessary in all cases with suspected lumbar spine injury..." This paper underscores the need to evaluate the entire spine in cases of motor-vehicle accidents, not just the cervical region. It may be cited when claims for lumbar radiographs are questioned in cases of children involved in car accidents.

Rachesky et al.[17] reported that on the cervical spine radiographs of children under 18 they examined, vehicular accidents accounted for 36% of radiographic abnormalities. It was further stated that clinical assessment of a complaint of neck pain or involvement in a vehicular accident with head trauma would have identified all cases of cervical spine injury.

Other authors have described aspects of cervical spine injuries in children involved in motor-vehicle accidents. Hill et al.[18] noted that 31% of the pediatric neck injuries reviewed were the result of motor-vehicle accidents. In younger children (under 8 years of age) subluxation was seen more frequently than fracture. Agran[19] stated that non-crash vehicular events may cause injuries to children. Non-crash events discussed in this paper included sudden stops, swerves, turns, and movement of unrestrained children in the vehicle.

Roberts et al.[20] described a case where a child involved in a motor-vehicle accident sustained a "whiplash" injury resulting in immediate neck and back pain. Neurobehavioral abnormalities increased in the two-year period following the accident. Four years after the accident, symptoms persisted. Position emission tomography (PET scan) demonstrated evidence of brain dysfunction.

The clinical manifestations of pediatric cervical spine injury may be diverse. Biedermann[21] stated that a wide range of pediatric symptomatology may result from suboccipital strain. The disorders reported include fever of unknown origin, loss of appetite, sleeping disorders, asymmetric motor patterns, and alterations of posture. Maigne[22] stated that trauma to the cervical spine and head can cause such problems as headaches, vestibular troubles, auditory problems and psychic disturbances. Gutmann[23] discussed the diverse array of signs and symptoms which can occur as a result of biomechanical dysfunction in the cervical spine. Others have also reported various pathoneurophysiological changes in children,[24-31] as well as reduction of pathology following chiropractic care.[29,31-41,44] In the chiropractic literature, Clow[42] published a paper addressing pediatric cervical acceleration/deceleration injuries.

Two peer reviewed journals, Chiropractic Pediatrics and the Journal of Clinical Chiropractic Pediatrics are being published to disseminate critically reviewed papers in this field. Additionally, courses in pediatrics are offered at the professional and postgraduate levels at accredited chiropractic colleges and by the International Chiropractic Pediatric Association.

The pediatric case history and physical examination necessarily differ in content and scope from those of adult patients. Even taking into consideration the difference between the two populations, however, a recent quasi meta-analysis reveals an extremely low risk for chiropractic pediatric patients receiving adjustments.[43]

9   Patient Safety

RECOMMENDATION

Patient safety encompasses the entire spectrum of care offered by the chiropractor. Consequently, it is important to define at the onset, the nature of the practice as well as the limits of care to be offered. Minimally this should include a "Terms of Acceptance" document between the practitioner and the patient. Additionally, all aspects of clinical practice should be carefully chosen to offer the patient the greatest advantage with the minimum of risk.

Rating: Established

Evidence: E, L

Commentary

Patient safety is assured by more than the practitioner's causing no harm. Since every consumer of health care is ultimately responsible for his/her own health choices, patient safety is also a matter of the availability of accurate and adequate information with which the patient must make these choices. The patient's expectations should be consistent with the provider's goals. If the patient perceives those goals as anything different, proper and safe choices cannot be assured. Thus, it is important to recognize that chiropractic is a limited, primary profession which contributes to health by addressing the safe detection, location, and correction or stabilization of vertebral subluxation(s). It is important that the chiropractor take the steps necessary to foster proper patient perception and expectation of the practitioner's professional goals and responsibilities. It is within this context that patient safety is addressed in this chapter.

A "Terms of Acceptance" is the recorded written informed consent agreement between a chiropractor and the patient. This document provides the patient with disclosure of the responsibilities of the chiropractor and limits of chiropractic, and the reasonable benefit to be expected. This enables the patient to make an informed choice either to engage the services of the chiropractor, aware of the intended purpose of the care involved, or not to engage those services if the proposed goals are not acceptable or not desired. This embodies the responsibility of assuring

138

patient safety by not providing false or misleading promises, claims or pretenses to the patient.[1-7]

Professional Referral: Professional referral requires authority and competence to acquire accurate information concerning matters within the scope and practice of the professional to whom a referral is made. There are two types of professional referrals made by chiropractors:

(A) Intraprofessional referral: Chiropractors, by virtue of their professional objective, education, and experience, have authority and competence to make direct referrals within the scope and practice of chiropractic. Such a referral may be made when the attending chiropractor is not able to address the specific chiropractic needs of a particular patient. Under these circumstances, the chiropractor may refer the patient directly to or consult with another chiropractor better suited by skill, experience or training to address the patient's chiropractic needs.

(B) Interprofessional referral: In the course of patient assessment and the delivery of chiropractic care, a practitioner may encounter findings which are outside his/her professional and/or legal scope, responsibility, or authority to address. The chiropractor has a responsibility to report such findings to the patient, and record their existence. Additionally, the patient should be advised that it is outside the responsibility and scope of chiropractic to offer advice, assessment or significance, diagnosis, prognosis, or treatment for said findings and that, if the patient chooses, he/she may consult with another provider, while continuing to have his/her chiropractic needs addressed.

Rare case reports of adverse events following spinal "manipulation" exist in the literature. However, scientific evidence of a causal relationship between such adverse events and the "manipulation" is lacking. Furthermore, spinal adjustment and spinal manipulation are not synonymous terms.

In the case of strokes purportedly associated with "manipulation," the panel noted significant shortcomings in the literature. A summary of the relevant literature follows:

*Lee[8] attempted to obtain an estimate of how often practicing neurologists in California encountered unexpected strokes, myelopathies, or radiculopathies following "chiropractic manipulation." Neurologists were asked the number of patients evaluated over the preceding two years who suffered a neurological complication within 24 hours of receiving "chiropractic manipulation." Fifty-five strokes were reported. The author stated, "Patients, physicians, and chiropractors should be aware of the risk of neurologic complications associated with chiropractic manipulation." No support was offered to substantiate the premise that a causal relationship existed between the stroke and the event(s) of the preceding 24 hours.

*In a letter to the editor of the Journal of Manipulative and Physiological Therapeutics, Myler[9] wrote, "I was curious how the risk of fatal stroke after cervical manipulation, placed at 0.00025%[10] compared with the risk of (fatal) stroke in the general population of the United States." According to data obtained from the National Center for Health Statistics, the mortality rate from stroke in the general population was calculated to be 0.00057%. If these data are correct, the risk of a fatal stroke following "cervical manipulation" is less than half the risk of fatal stroke in the general population.

*Jaskoviak[11] reported that not a single case of vertebral artery stroke occurred in approximately five million cervical "manipulations" at the National College of Chiropractic Clinic from 1965 to 1980.

*Osteopathic authors Vick, et al.[12] reported that from 1923 to 1993, there were only 185 reports of injury associated with "several million treatments."

*Pistolese[13] has constructed a risk assessment for pediatric chiropractic patients. His findings covering approximately the last 30 years indicate a risk of a neurological and/or vertebrobasilar accident during a chiropractic visit about one in every 250,000,000 visits.

*An article in the "Back Letter"[14] noted that "In scientific terms, all these figures are rough guesses at best... There is currently no accurate data on the total number of cervical manipulations performed every year or the total number of complications. Both figures would be necessary to arrive at an accurate estimate. In addition, none of the studies in the medical literature adequately control for other risk factors and co-morbidities."

*Leboeuf-Yde et al.[15] suggested that there may be an over-reporting of "spinal manipulative therapy" related injuries. The authors reported cases involving two fatal strokes, a heart attack, a bleeding basilar aneurysm, paresis of an arm and a leg, and cauda equina syndrome which occurred in individuals who were considering chiropractic care, yet because of chance, did not receive it. Had these events been temporally related to a chiropractic office visit, they may have been inappropriately attributed to chiropractic care.

*In many cases of strokes attributed to chiropractic care, the "operator" was not a chiropractor at all. Terrett[16] observed that "manipulations" administered by Kung Fu practitioner, GPs, osteopaths, physiotherapists, a wife, a blind masseur, and an Indian barber were incorrectly attributed to chiropractors. As Terrett wrote, "The words chiropractic and chiropractor have been incorrectly used in numerous publications dealing with SMT injury by medical authors, respected medical journals and medical organizations. In many cases, this is not accidental; the authors had access to original reports that identified the practitioner involved as a non-chiropractor. The true incidence of such reporting cannot be determined. Such reporting adversely affects the reader's opinion of chiropractic and chiropractors."

*Another error made in these reports was failure to differentiate "cervical manipulation" from specific chiropractic adjustment. Klougart et al.[17] published risk estimates which revealed differences which were dependent upon the type of technique used by the chiropractor.

The panel found no competent evidence that specific chiropractic adjustments cause strokes. Although vertebrobasilar screening procedures are taught in chiropractic colleges, no reliable screening tests were identified which enable a chiropractor to identify patients who are at risk for stroke.

After examining twelve patients with dizziness reproduced by extension rotation and twenty healthy controls with Doppler ultrasound of the vertebral arteries, Cote, et al.[18] concluded, "We were unable to demonstrate that the extension-rotation test is a valid clinical screening procedure to detect decreased blood flow in the vertebral artery. The value of this test for screening patients at risk of stroke after cervical manipulation is questionable." Terrett[19] noted, "There is no evidence which suggests that positive tests have any correlation to future VBS (vertebrobasilar stroke) and SMT (spinal manipulative therapy)." Despite this lack of evidence, some have suggested that failure to employ such tests could place a chiropractor in a less defensible position should litigation ensue following a CVA.[20]

141

10   Professional Development

RECOMMENDATION

Continuing professional development, as in all responsible health professions, is a necessary component of maintaining a high standard for both the practitioner and the profession. Continuing development should be directed to areas germane to each individual practice, including but not limited to: credentialing, continuing education programs, participation in professional organizations, ethics forums, and legal issues.

Rating: Established
Evidence: E, L

Commentary

Continuing professional development is currently widely mandated by most licensing jurisdictions, or encouraged through most professional organizations. Perhaps the most compelling reason for advocating this type of on-going education is to afford practitioners the opportunity to keep abreast of current issues, techniques, and methods which serve to enhance patient care. The fact that most programs are conducted by individuals skilled in the topics presented, also provides a high ratio of quality information delivered in a relatively short period. Thus, professional development serves not only the practitioner, but ultimately benefits the patient through enhanced practice skills acquired in different areas by the chiropractor.[1-14]

In addition to formal postgraduate education courses, other opportunities for professional development may include:

- Reading scholarly journals
- Attending scientific symposia
- Participation in research
- Publication of clinical and scientific papers
- Audio and videocassette courses
- Teleclasses
- Distance education programs

Index

143